C-MASS

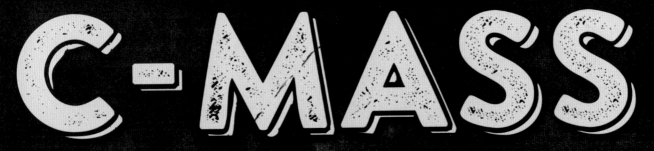

CALISTHENICS MASS:

HOW TO MAXIMIZE MUSCLE GROWTH USING BODYWEIGHT-ONLY TRAINING

PAUL "COACH" WADE
AUTHOR OF CONVICT CONDITIONING

C-MASS
CALISTHENICS MASS

PAUL "COACH" WADE

ISBN 10: 0-938045-74-1   ISBN 13: 978-0-938045-74-8
This edition first published in September, 2014
Printed in China

Book design and cover by Derek Brigham • www.dbrigham.com • bigd@dbrigham.com

— CONTENTS —

Dedicated to all the members of the PCC community.

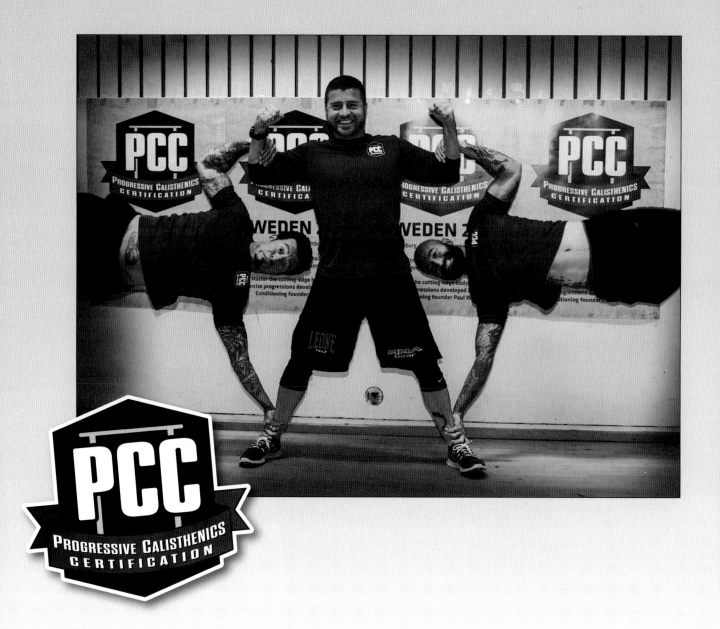

FOREWORD

This book began its life as an extensive two-part post on the Progressive Calisthenics Certification blog. The posts were titled *The Ten Commandments of Calisthenics Mass*. (I groove on numbers and regimented lists, in case ya hadn't noticed...the "Big Six", then Ten Steps, etc. A left-over of prison life, no doubt.)

After hundreds of questions and comments—many via email—it became clear that the theme had struck a nerve. This issue of muscle-gain and its relationship to calisthenics is a biggie, and it always has been. Folks had questions, new ideas, observations...in short, they wanted more than a couple of blog articles could deliver.

That's why I was prompted to write this book—*C-MASS*. It contains an edited and extended version of the original two articles, welded together for clarity and reference purposes. There is also a stack of new material added just for the book, including a chapter explaining the essence of bodyweight bodybuilding, a section on programming, bodypart training tips and a full FAQ guide to help with any troubleshooting, plus more.

This book is dedicated to the members of the PCC community who made it happen. If you get a kick out of this manual, hop on down to the PCC blog and make a comment or contribution. Join the fastest-growing elite bodyweight training community on planet Earth.

I hope to see ya there, muscles!

Paul "Coach" Wade 2014

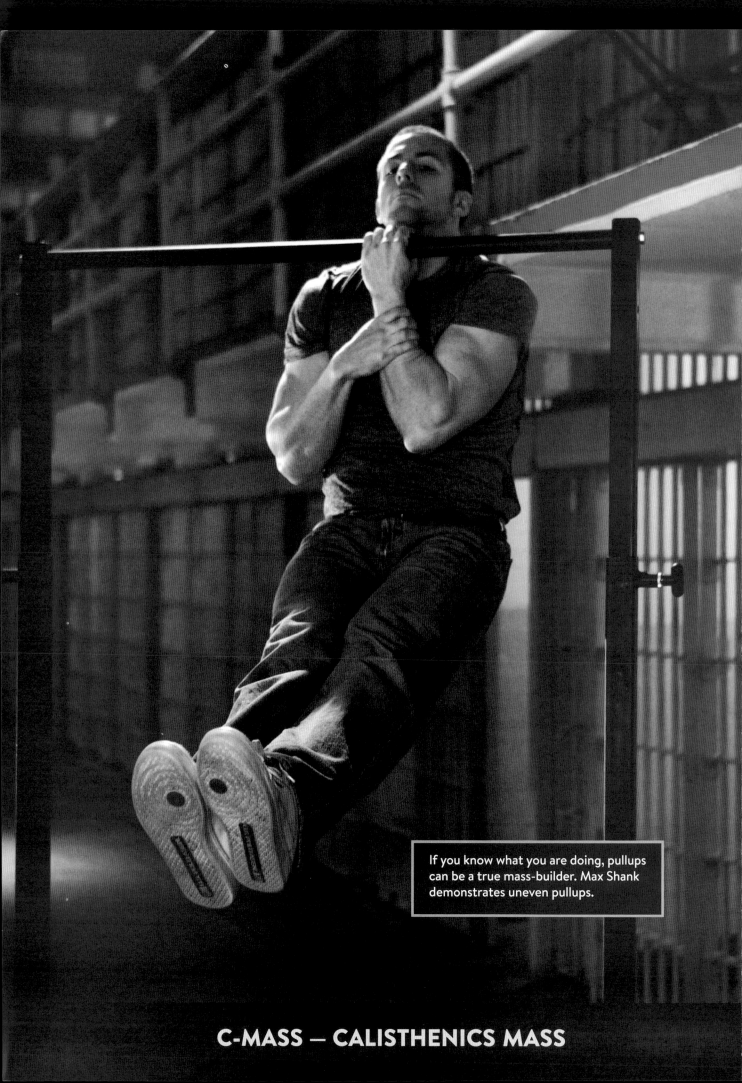

If you know what you are doing, pullups can be a true mass-builder. Max Shank demonstrates uneven pullups.

C-MASS — CALISTHENICS MASS

1

BODYWEIGHT MUSCLE? NO PROBLEM!

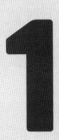n my mind, there is a picture. It is a hot summer day in San Quentin. I'm in the yard, queuing to use the pullup bar. I can't remember the year—it was so long ago, many of you reading this will not have even been born. But what I can remember was the guy in front of me—*Dixon*. Dixon was an inmate so wide, you couldn't see behind the man in a hallway. His lats were so damn thick, I wondered how he could even keep his arms by his side. His deltoids were genuine spheres of muscle, so large and well-shaped that they looked as if they'd been sculpted on. His triceps were particularly awesome; when he raised his arms they hung down like glistening shark's bellies, solid curves of human steel.

Dixon wasn't a juicer. We all knew who used steroids inside, and back in the day there were fewer than you might believe, if you saw the physiques. And Dixon never *touched* a weight or a machine—certainly not to build muscle. He purchased his incredible muscles through *bodyweight work,* and he paid for them in pain.

Dixon wasn't alone. I met many, many dudes who built *phenomenal* amounts of natural muscle mass—often going from thin and stringy—using bodyweight-only methods. You can do it, too. How would you like to level-up your physique? I'm talking about:

- Adding 20-30 pounds of solid muscle
- Reshaping your arms with 2-3 inches of beef
- Tripling the size of your pecs and lats
- Thickening and hardening your abdominal wall into a classic six-pack
- Throwing a thick, healthy vein onto your biceps
- Generating hard, sculpted quads and hamstrings like an Olympic sprinter
- Building true "diamond" calves

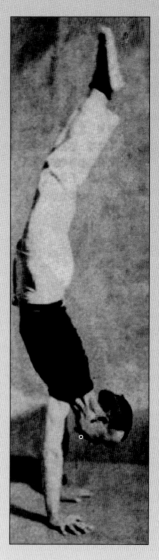
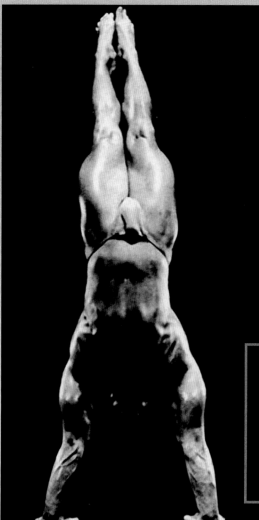

There is so much *artificial* inflation of muscle size, so much nonsense talked about measurements in modern bodybuilding, that to some of you these kind of gains maybe seem modest. Trust me—they ain't. If you can achieve these gains, you will be head and shoulders above the next 99% of natural bodybuilders, who very rarely achieve any noticeable results at all.

The handstands look identical, but they are practiced in very different ways. Professor Paulinetti (*left*) became one of the strongest bodyweight athletes in history. Ed Theriault (*right*) became Mr Canada.

WHY AREN'T MANY BODYWEIGHT ATHLETES AS BIG AS THEY ARE STRONG?

When I was behind bars, it's safe to say that most cons knew that serious, hardcore bodyweight training could build serious, hardcore muscles on a brother—no matter what his starting point. It saddens me to say it, but on the outside, this is not the case. Bodyweight strength training is not typically associated with huge muscles in the modern fitness world. This is coz you can find loads of bodyweight enthusiasts who can perform phenomenal feats of strength—one-arm handstands, human flags, planches, etc.—despite looking fairly "normal". Skinny, even.

How is that that bodyweight training has made these guys so strong, so fit, but not as massive as bodybuilders?

The answer has to do with *training methodology*. Generally speaking—I'm paraphrasing here, kid—there are TWO types of resistance training, both at different ends of the spectrum. The first is *nervous system* training. The second is *muscular system* training.

Believe it or not, these two kinds of bodyweight training are poles apart...and they give *radically* different results! To best understand the differences between the two, check out the table below.

	NERVOUS SYSTEM TRAINING	MUSCULAR SYSTEM TRAINING
ADAPTATION	The nervous system adapts by reconfiguring: the cells communicate more *efficiently*	The muscular system adapts by adding extra chemical energy: the muscle cells swell and become *larger*
METHOD	Pick an exercise you find challenging and attempt to perform it *perfectly* as *many times* as possible	Pick a difficult exercise, then perform it for *as long as you can* until your muscles are drained
EFFORT	Stay "fresh". If you push too hard your form will not be perfect and you will exhaust yourself	Push as hard as you can during your work sets. Your goal is to exhaust your muscles, to force them to adapt
NO. OF REPS	As the exercise is challenging, you will only be able to perform a small number of reps: 1-5 (ideally 1-3)	For the muscles to be optimally drained of their chemical energy, you need more reps: 6-20 (ideally around 10)
NO. OF SETS	Since you wish to perform the technique many times (with low reps) you need lots of sets	The muscles can be drained very quickly and efficiently with a low number of sets, provided the reps are high enough
FREQUENCY	The nervous system reconfigures quickly—since you stay fresh, you can even train multiple times daily	The muscular system needs time to heal and increase cellular size. Add in plenty of rest and off-days
PSYCHOLOGY	You approach your training sessions as "practice" periods. Try to develop *skill*	You approach your training sessions as challenging "workouts". Try to push yourself *hard*

The basic differences between nervous and muscular system training

Modern bodyweight students tend to adhere to methodologies built around *nervous system* training. They make their nervous systems much more efficient at utilizing their muscles. They develop superior coordination, balance and spatial skills. Because of this, they don't require significantly larger muscles to be able to perform their feats of bodyweight strength.

Much of this training philosophy has been drawn from gymnastics. Gymnasts really don't *want* huge muscles—they primarily train their nervous systems. (Yes, I know that some gymnasts are extremely muscular...but they don't specifically train to get that way. If they did, they'd be even bigger!)

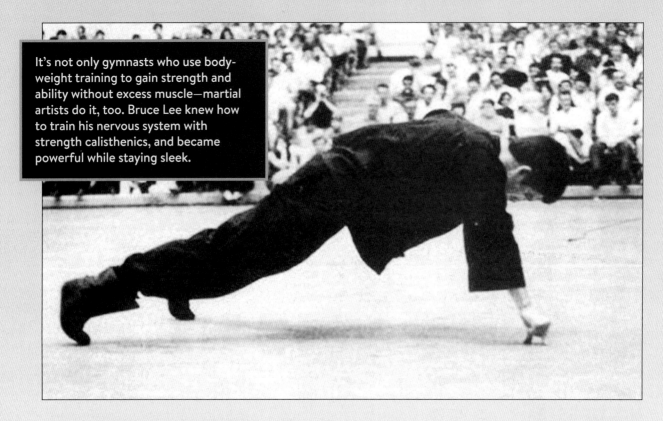

It's not only gymnasts who use bodyweight training to gain strength and ability without excess muscle—martial artists do it, too. Bruce Lee knew how to train his nervous system with strength calisthenics, and became powerful while staying sleek.

Now, don't get me wrong...I am a *huge* admirer of this kind of nervous system training, and have used it extensively myself. But if you really want to explode your muscle growth, you should not be training your *nervous system*—you should be training your *muscular system*. I have seen lots of athletes—those wanting to size-up—apply themselves to bodyweight training, only to sabotage their efforts by utilizing the common methods of nervous system training. They get stronger and more capable at bodyweight exercises, but don't gain much in the way of size. Then, six months later, they quit, and tell everybody; *yeah, bodyweight is good for strength, but it won't put on much size.*

Bullshit!

They were doing it wrong! If they had used an approach designed to train their *muscles*—as opposed to primarily training their *nervous system*—they would have gained all the muscle they wanted. If size is your goal, you gotta shift your training away from nervous system-style work to pure muscular work. Stop training like a *gymnast*, and start training like a *bodybuilder*. Gymnasts are masters at building bodyweight strength and ability, but bodybuilders know all about building big muscles. They understand what it means to train the muscular system.

So, next question: what does it mean to train your "muscles"? To make things easy, I've boiled muscular training down into Ten Commandments. If you want to build some *real* muscle over the next few months, forget the typical nervous system methods and knuckle down to applying these ten ideas.

You WILL NOT believe the results.

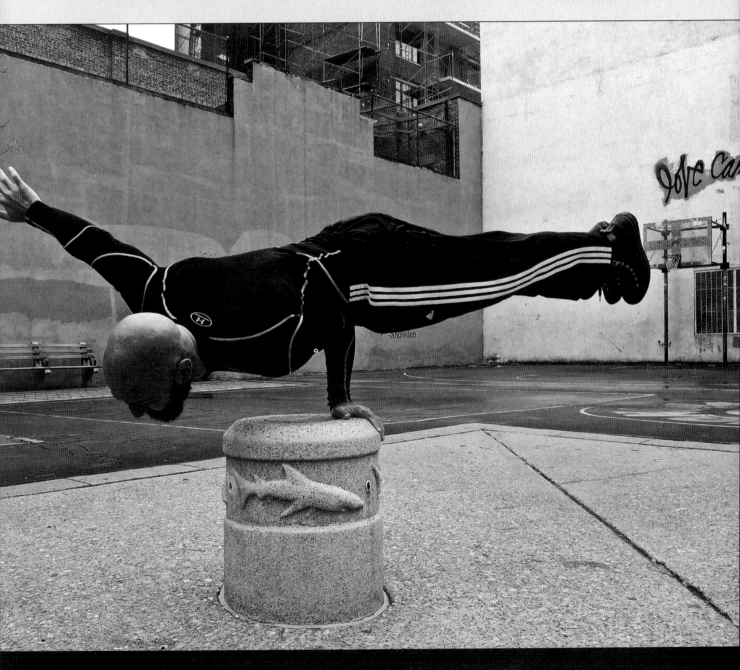

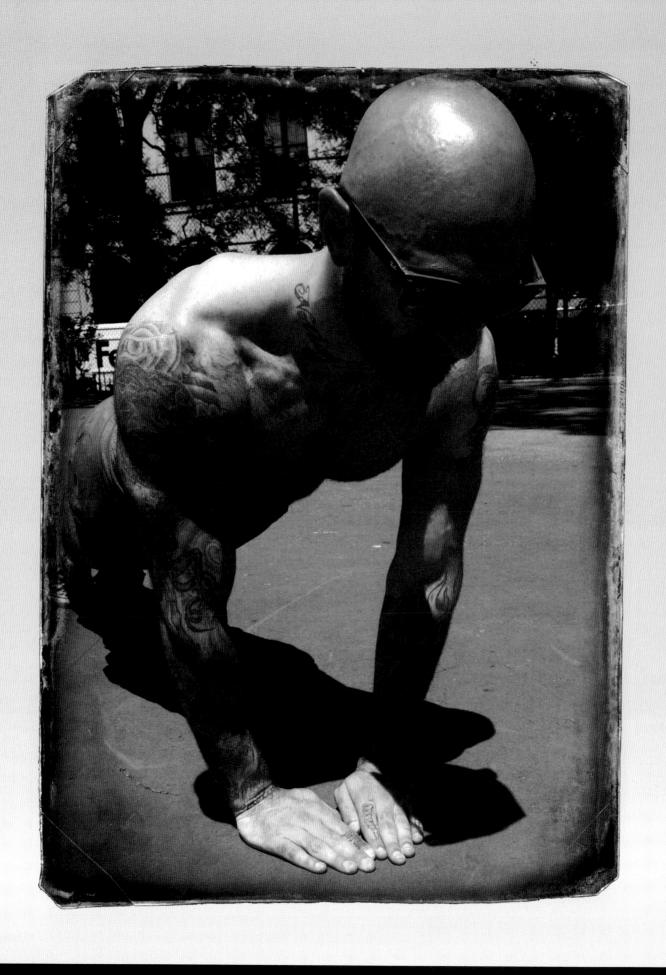

C-MASS — CALISTHENICS MASS

2

THE TEN COMMANDMENTS OF CALISTHENICS MASS

COMMANDMENT I: EMBRACE REPS!

These days, low reps, high sets and low fatigue are the "in" methodology. Why low reps with low fatigue? Coz it's great for building *skill*. If you want to get really good at a movement—be it a handstand or an elbow lever—the key is to train your *nervous system*. That means performing an exercise perfectly plenty of times, to beat the ideal movement pattern into your "neural map". The best way to achieve this is to do a few low reps—not hard or long enough to burn out or get too tired—then rest for a bit and try again. Wash, rinse, repeat. This is typically how very lean, low-weight bodyweight guys train to get hugely strong but without adding too much muscle. It's a phenomenal way to drill efficient motion-pathways into your nervous system, while keeping fresh. Like I say, it's ideal for training a *skill*.

But for stacks of jacked up muscle? Sorry, this method just won't cut it. Muscle isn't built by training the *nervous system*. It's built by training the MUSCLE! And for this, you need reps, kiddo. Lovely, lovely, reps.

To cut a long story short, you build big muscles by draining the chemical energy in your muscle cells. Over time, your body responds to this threat by accumulating greater and greater stores of chemical energy in those cells. This makes them swell, and voila—bigger muscles. But to trigger this extra storage, you gotta exhaust the chemical energy in those cells. This can only be done by *hard, sustained work*. Gentle work won't do it—if the exercise is too low in intensity, the energy will come from fatty acids and other stores, rather than the precious muscle cells. Intermittent work—low reps, rest, repeat—won't do it either, because the chemical energy in the cells rapidly regenerates when you rest, meaning stores never get dangerously low enough for the body to say "uh-oh—better stockpile bigger banks of this energy!"

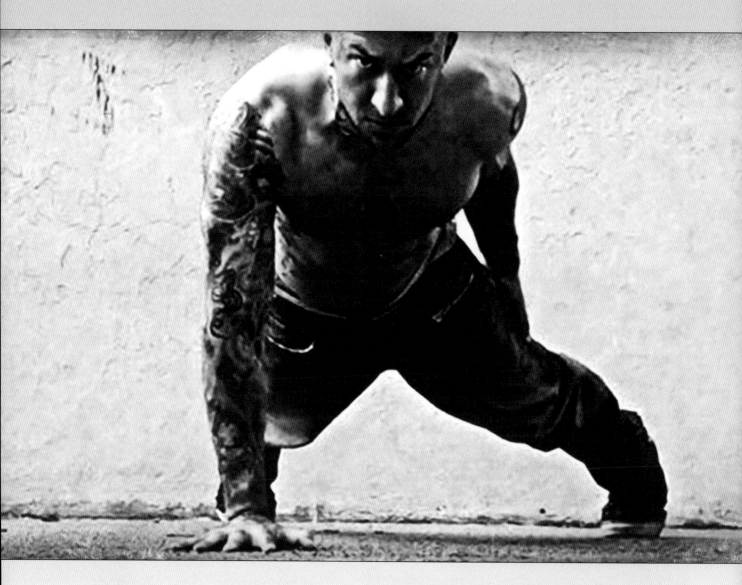

The best way to exhaust the energy in your muscles is through tough, grit-yer-teeth, continuous reps. Learn to love 'em. For huge gains, temporarily drop the single, double, and triple reps. Definitely start looking at reps over five. Six to eight is great. Double figures are even better. Twelve to fifteen is another muscle-building range. I've met very strong guys training with low reps for years who couldn't build a quarter inch on their arms. They switched to performing horizontal pulls for sets of twenty reps, and gained two inches per arm in a *single month*! These kind of gains aren't uncommon on *Convict Conditioning*, due to the insistence that you pay your dues with higher reps. They work!

COMMANDMENT II: WORK HARD!

This Commandment directly follows from the last one. Using low reps, keeping fresh, and taking lots of rest between sets is a fairly easy way to train. But pushing through continuous rep after rep on hard exercises is much, *much* tougher. The higher the reps, the harder it gets.

Your muscles will burn and scream at you to quit. (That "burning" is your chemical energy stores being incinerated for fuel, which is exactly what you want!) Your heart-rate will shoot through the roof; you will tremble, sweat, and feel systemic stress. You may even feel nauseous.

Good! You are doing something *right*!

Like I say, the current trend is towards easy sets, keeping fresh, working on skill. These days you don't "work out", you *practice*. "Working " and "pushing yourself"....these are filthy terms in gyms today. They are considered old-fashioned, from outta the seventies and eighties. (Remember those decades? When drug-free dudes in the gym actually had some f***ing *muscle*?) I mean Christ, some coaches take this philosophy so far that you'd think if an athlete went to "failure", their goddam balls would drop off. Jesus!

Sure, I don't recommend going to complete failure on bodyweight exercise—at least, most of the time. I'd prefer it if you left a *little* energy in your body after a set to control your movements, and maybe defend yourself if you have to. But that doesn't mean you shouldn't work hard. Damn hard.

Far from destroying you physically, brutal effort—when moderated by plenty of rest and sleep—causes the body to release testosterone, growth hormone, endorphins, and plenty of other goodies Mother Nature always intended to reward Her hunters and warriors with.

So accept the challenge. Balls, wall—together, okay? Don't ever be afraid to push yourself into new zones of pain and effort if you want to get bigger. I have seen *twigs* turned into *oaks* this way, and you can do it too—I believe in you!

Whatever modern coaches may say, don't be afraid of pushing yourself.

COMMANDMENT III:
USE SIMPLE, COMPOUND EXERCISES!

Again, this Commandment is related to the two which have gone before. If you are going to push yourself *hard* on *moderate-to-high reps*, the exercises you are doing can't be complex, high-skill exercises. If handstands and elbow levers cause you to concentrate to balance, you can't overload using them—your form would collapse (and so would you) before you were pushing yourself hard enough to drain your muscles.

So if you want to work with high-skill exercises, use the low reps/keep fresh/high sets philosophy. But if you want to get *swole*, you need relatively low skill exercises—this is what I mean by "simple" exercises. "Simple" doesn't mean "easy". Doing twenty perfect one-arm pushups is "simple"—it ain't easy!

Stick to exercises you can pour a huge amount of muscular effort into, without wasting nervous energy on factors like balance, coordination, gravity, body placement, etc. *Dynamic* exercises—where you go up and down—are generally far better than *static holds*, because they typically require less concentration and they drain the muscle cells more rapidly.

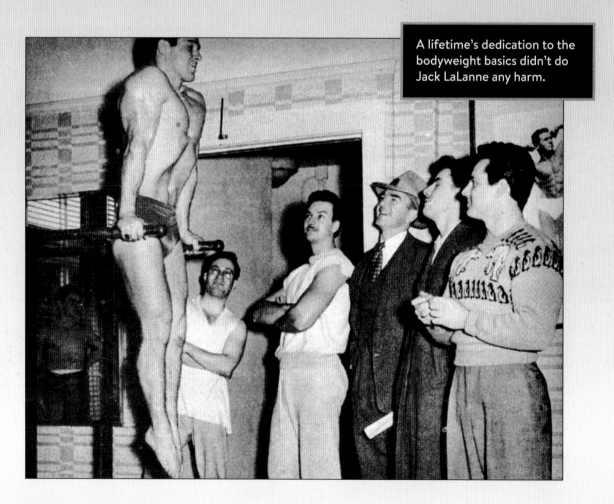

A lifetime's dedication to the bodyweight basics didn't do Jack LaLanne any harm.

The best dynamic exercises are *compound* exercises, which involve multiple muscle groups at once. Not only are these simpler—the body works as a whole, which is more natural—but you are getting a bigger bang for your buck by working different muscles at the same time. (No weak links for you, Daniel-san.) For example, focus on:

- Pullups
- Bodyweight squats, pistols and shrimp squats
- Pushups
- Australian pullup variations

- Dips
- Bridges
- Handstand pushups (against a wall—lower skill, more effort)
- Leg raises

All of these movements can be made increasingly difficult to suit your muscle-building rep range (see Commandment V). There are *no* excuses for not kicking your own ass, here.

Don't get me wrong. This is not to say that skill-based techniques—like elbow levers and handstands—don't have a place in your program. They are valuable exercises and are taught extensively as part of the PCC curriculum. But using them exclusively for muscle gain is definitely a big mistake. Throw in simple, compound moves and watch those muscles sprout like never before!

COMMANDMENT IV: LIMIT SETS!

This is another pretty controversial suggestion—but, as always, it flows from the previous Commandments perfectly. Why? Well, if you are hitting your body with hard exercises, and pouring that effort into enough reps to completely exhaust the muscles, why would you need to perform lots of sets?

Depleting your muscle cells beyond the point your body is comfortable with is what causes the biological "survival trigger" that tells your body to add more energy (i.e., extra muscle) for next time. That's all you need to do. Once you have pulled that trigger and told your body to make more muscle...why keep pulling the trigger, again and again? It's a waste of time and energy—worse in fact, because it damages the muscles further and eats into your recovery time. In the words of infamous exercise ideologist, Mike Mentzer:

> *"You can take a stick of dynamite and tap it with a pencil all day and it's not going to go off.*
> *But hit it once with a hammer and 'BANG'—it will go off!"*
>
> — Mike Mentzer

Many folks disagree with Mentzer's training philosophy—I don't agree with all of it—but he certainly nailed it when he said this. The biological switch for muscle growth needs to be triggered with a hammer, not a f***ing pencil. One hard, focused, exhausting set on a compound exercise is worth more than twenty, thirty half-hearted sets.

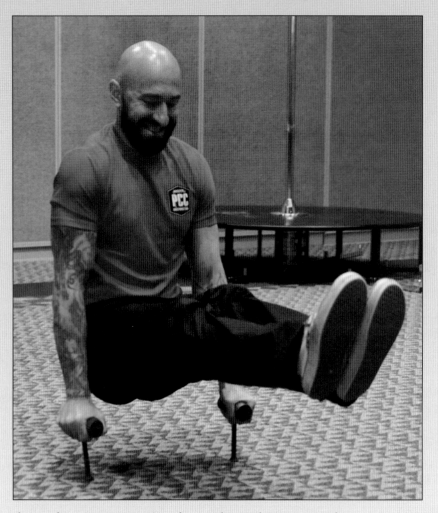

I usually advise folks looking for maximum growth to perform *two* hard sets per exercise, following a proper warm-up. Growth will happen with one set, but two sets feels like a belt-and-braces approach. I sometimes advise more sets for beginners, but this not for growth—it's to help them get more experience with a movement. It's practice, basically. Once you know how to perform an exercise properly, two hard sets is all you need.

Many eager trainees ask me if they should perform more sets. The trouble is, adding sets does not encourage hard, high-performance training—*just the opposite*. Once you are doing five, six sets, one of two things happens; either you give your all and your last sets are pathetic compared to the first couple of sets, or you pace yourself, making *all* the sets weaker than they would be otherwise. Neither of these situations will promote extra growth. They just hinder recovery and increase the risk of injury.

Avoid "volume creep". Training *hard* is very different from training *long*—in fact, the two are mutually exclusive. Keep workouts short and sharp and reap the rewards, kemosabe!

COMMANDMENT V: FOCUS ON PROGRESS— AND UTILIZE A TRAINING JOURNAL!

Believe it or not, there are some folks who focus on the previous four Commandments—they exhaust their muscles, work hard, use the best exercises and put all their energy into a small number of sets—and still make very little in the way of meaningful gains. This is true even if they train year-to-year. Maybe this is you—I'm sure you know folks like this.

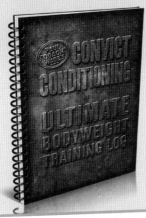

Why does this travesty happen?

Is it genetics? Is it the fact that they train without steroids? Is it because their balls haven't dropped? Is it the fact that their gym doesn't sell the latest superbolictastic high-sugar/high toxicity supps, bro?!

None of the above, Jim. To discover the true reason, read the following excerpt from the *Convict Conditioning Ultimate Bodyweight Log*:

If making progress in training is so simple, why do so few wannabe athletes ever achieve a good level of strength and muscle—let alone a *great* level?

The answer is that few trainees take advantage of the *windows of opportunity* their training presents to them. You see, when you work out, your body adapts to cope with the stress, but it only adapts a tiny little bit; this is especially true once you get beyond the beginner stages of training. Improvements are small—maybe you add a rep here; you improve your form there; you increase your recovery time somewhere else. Over months and years, however, these small increases eventually add up to very big increases. This is how seemingly "inhuman" athletes double and triple their strength, add inches of solid muscle, and transform themselves into superior physical beings.

Sadly, since most trainees aren't paying attention to those tiny changes, they never build on them the way they should. These little weekly changes are actually *windows of opportunity*. If you could increase your strength by just 1% every week, you could more than double your strength in just two years. But most trainees never get anywhere close to doubling their strength, because they aren't keeping track of their training accurately. They fail to recognize that 1% adaptation—the rep here, the improved form there. If you miss these *little* improvements, how can you build on them to make *big* improvements?

1% is actually a pretty small target to hit. When you rely on memory, instinct or feeling—as so many trainers do—to hit this target, it becomes very *fuzzy*. (Which is the last thing you want from small target, right?) Writing your progress down in a log makes this small target clear and easy to see. It makes it quantifiable. Athletes who begin writing simple log entries of their workouts find they suddenly know what they need to do to progress every single time they work out. They never miss that tiny 1%.

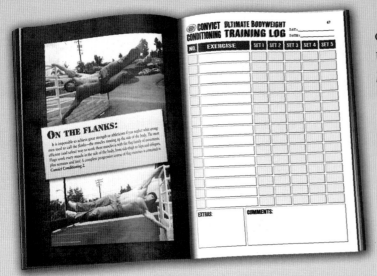

There you have it. In reality, the previous four Commandments are worthless unless you harness them all to make *progress*—week to week, month to month, year to year. It doesn't matter how seemingly insignificant these improvements are. Over the months and years they add up. In a nutshell, the "secret" to drug-free muscle and strength gain is to become acutely aware of the tiny improvements in your performance, and build on them on a regular basis. The best way to make this happen is to keep a training journal.

Anyone who is familiar with my writings knows that I am a *huge* believer in keeping a training log to determine progress—*especially where muscle-building is the goal*. It always amazes me that folks will spend hundreds of bucks on worthless supplements, but won't take a few minutes to keep a log of their training. It's ironic, coz *a simple training log, used correctly, will do more for your physique than any over-the-counter supplement on the planet*. I could write a whole article on the benefits of keeping a log…monitoring progress, contemplating feedback, mastering training science, improving workout mindfulness…the list goes on!

I put together the CC training log because a lot of athletes complained to me that most commercial logs weren't geared towards bodyweight. The log means a lot to me, and I put a *ton* of advice and cool photos in there. I'm real proud of the journal for many reasons, but I'm honestly not trying to sell you anything here. You don't *have* to buy *this* log to keep a journal…the beauty of calisthenics is that you don't *have* to buy anything!

Just get your hands on a cheap notepad, or use your computer. But please, do it. Do it for old Coach!

COMMANDMENT VI:
YOU GROW WHEN YOU REST. SO REST!

Again—the issue of *rest* ("training frequency" for you guys with a better vocabulary than me) immediately follows on from the previous idea of *progress*.

Let me ask you a simple question. If you *really* wanted to improve on your last workout—add that rep, tighten up your form—how would you want to approach that workout?

Would you want to be tired, weary, beat-up?

No! That's nuts! Obviously you'd want to be as well-rested, as fresh as possible, to tear into your workout with as much energy as you could get, to break some records, increase your reps, improve your personal best!

It sounds like a dumb question. *Of course* you'd want to be as fresh, as rested as possible if you really wanted to give your all and maximize your muscle-growth stimulation, right?

Yet this is exactly the *opposite* of what most wannabe bodybuilders do. Being brainwashed by the muscle rags—typically by trying to copy the programs of drugged-up steroid junkies, who can get away with training like pussies and working out seven times a day—they desperately try to deplete any mental and hormonal energy they have by training more and more often. Some of these guys are training the body hard four times a week...then they wonder why they aren't improving!

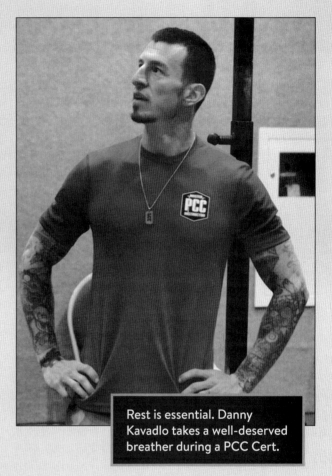

Rest is essential. Danny Kavadlo takes a well-deserved breather during a PCC Cert.

You don't need to be Kojak to know why they aren't improving. You don't need a PhD in molecular myology to know why they aren't improving. They are *tired*. Their muscles haven't had a chance to rest and heal, let alone recover and increase their size and strength. I admire the willpower of folks who are constantly working out, even when they are spinning their wheels—I've done it too. Some of it comes down to the glamor of training; we become so seduced by the idea of the exercises, we forget that we are tearing our muscles down when we train. We have forgotten that one simple, ancient muscle-building fact—*your muscles grow when you rest, not when you train.*

How much rest you need for optimal performance depends on your age, your constitution, your training experience, your other activities, etc. But I can give you a few general pointers:

• Working any muscle more than twice a week is usually a mistake if you want to gain size.

• How often you *train* doesn't matter a s***—how often you make *progress* is what matters.

• Working a muscle hard once a week—and actually making progress—is better than working it four times per week and going backwards.

• Never train any muscle hard two days in a row.

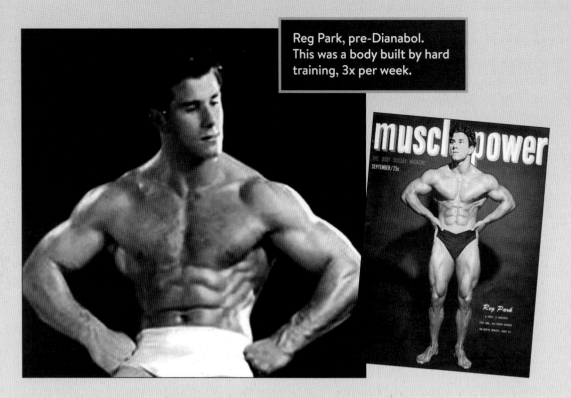

Reg Park, pre-Dianabol. This was a body built by hard training, 3x per week.

- Old school bodybuilders like Steve Reeves and Reg Park became huge by training—*hard*—only three days per week. To this day, many of the most massive powerlifters only train three days per week. The idea that you need to train every day (or several times per day) to maximize your potential is bullshit.

- Bigger muscles typically take longer to recover than smaller muscles.

- If a muscle group is sore, don't train it!

- Muscular training also depletes the hormonal and energy systems. If you feel low, tired or lacking energy, add another day or two of rest into your program—even if your muscles feel good.

- Always take *at least* two days off per week, for maximum muscle gain—unless you are performing very low volume workouts. Even then, three or four days off per week is probably better.

- The ultimate arbiter of a bodybuilding program is *progress*—in muscle size, but also in performance. If you are working hard but your reps aren't increasing, add another rest day.

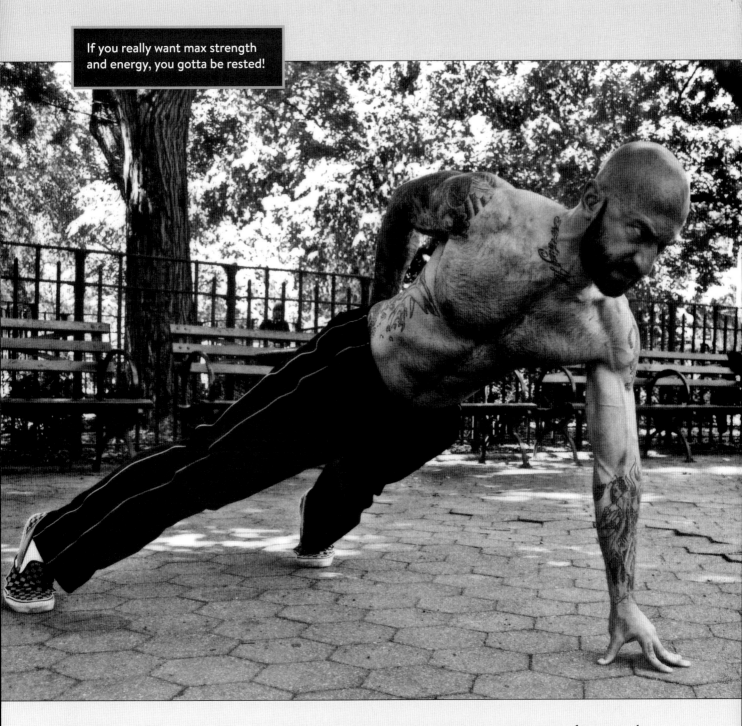

If you really want max strength and energy, you gotta be rested!

The bottom line: to build extra muscle you must continue to improve your performance by cranking out a greater workload over a small number of sets. To do this, your muscles (and your body) need to be *rested*. Rest is a bigger piece of the puzzle than most athletes ever realize—as a result, they never even come close to their full potential.

COMMANDMENT VII: QUIT EATING "CLEAN" THE WHOLE TIME!

Ah, we're on to nutrition now, boys and girls. My views on nutrition are so far from the norm that I even get snubbed at a George Zimmerman fundraiser. I can feel panties bunching with hatred and rage even as I write this. It's a great feeling—so let's keep going, huh?

Read a copy of any of the muscle or fitness based rags on the newsstands, and you'd think the perfect muscle meal was chicken breast with some broccoli—and hey, don't forget some supplements thrown in on the side. Washed down with plenty of water.

Crock. Of. S**t.

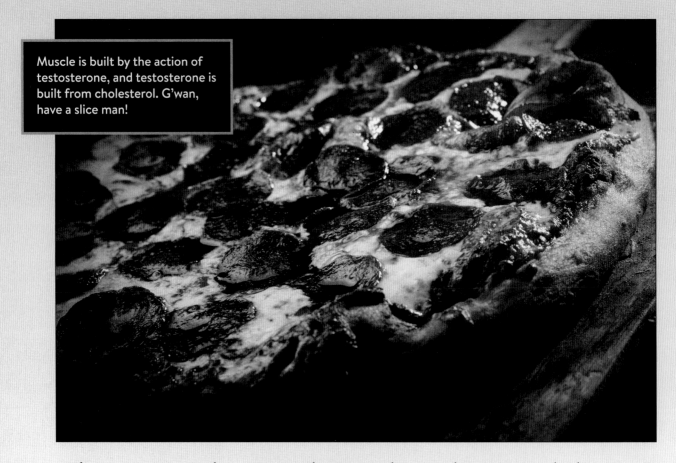

Muscle is built by the action of testosterone, and testosterone is built from cholesterol. G'wan, have a slice man!

If you are trying to pack on some muscle, eating junk now and again is not only okay, it's positively *anabolic*. In **Convict Conditioning 2**, I wrote about the prison diet, and described how some very muscular, very strong athletes maintained incredible physiques on diets that—to the mainstream fitness world—would be considered totally inadequate, on many counts. Let me tell you, if those guys could get their hands on a little junk every day, they would bite your arms off for it! They knew it fuelled the fires of growth.

One of the biggest sensations in the modern bodybuilding world is a guy who—these days, any-how—is known as *Kali Muscle*. Kali is 5'10" and weighs over 250lbs—with abs. Despite his bodyweight, Kali learned his trade in San Quentin, a prison culture surrounded by calisthenics athletes, and he can still perform impressive bodyweight feats like muscle-ups and the human flag. Kali says that he really began growing when he was in jail and began filling his body with "dirty" high-carb foods like Dunkin' Stix, Honey Buns, ramen and tuna spread. He says the effect these high calorie "junk" foods had on his skinny body was so profound, that he rejected offers of steroids during his prison years. He didn't need them.

Kali isn't crazy. His words are the truth. This idea—that the odd "junk" item is good for your training—is not a new one. Many of the old-time strongmen thrived on food that is considered crap today. The Saxon brothers ate cakes and drank beer as a daily staple of their diet. John Grimek used to drive around with oversized Hershey bars in his glove box, for emergencies.

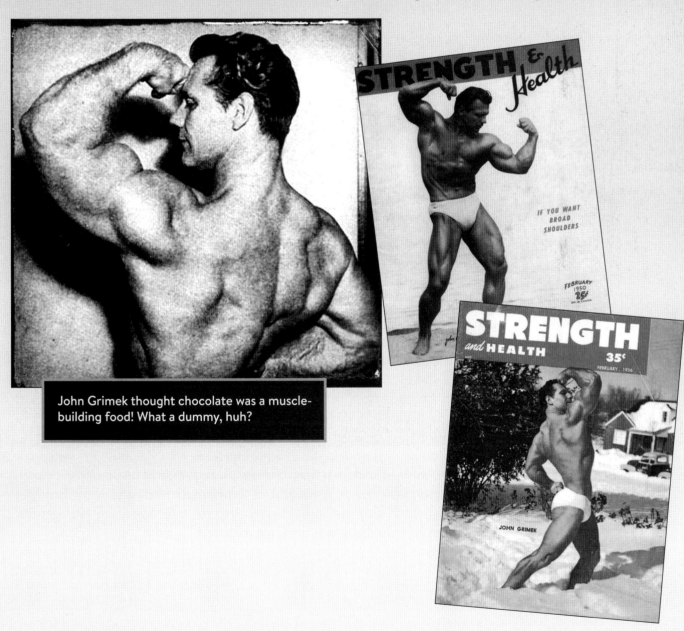

John Grimek thought chocolate was a muscle-building food! What a dummy, huh?

And throw some fatty stuff in there too, willya? Quit avoiding *real* "muscle foods" like red meat, egg yolks, ham, cheese and sausage. I have to laugh when I see skinny guys throwing thousands of bucks of amino acids and whey shakes down their necks, in a hopeless effort to get big. What the supplement companies (and their bitches, the fitness magazines) will never tell you is a basic fact known by *every endocrinologist on the planet*—testosterone (remember that? The muscle-building hormone?) is synthesized from *cholesterol*. That's right...without taking in enough cholesterol from high-fat foods, your body cannot create testosterone, and it cannot build muscle.

Vegans are always moaning that meat is full of pathogens and the like, but—far from killing us off—recent studies show that red meat might be what's responsible for our species' abnormally long life-spans. Our hungry ancestors literally adapted to slabs of meat, building super-immunity in the process.

I'm not saying you should act like a fat pig and eat junk all day (although maybe you should if you can't gain weight). If you want to get big you should eat a balanced, regulated diet. But eating "clean" the whole time will only hurt your gains. Throw in a little "junk" every day if you expect to get *swole*.

Go have that burger and a Twinkie. A couple hours later, you'll have the best workout of your life. You might even grow.

COMMANDMENT VIII: SLEEP MORE!

Since *Convict Conditioning* first came out, I've been deluged by a lot of questions about *prison athletes*. It's a subject folks—especially dudes—really seem interested in. How is it that prison athletes seem to gain and maintain so much dense muscle, when guys on the outside—who are taking supplements and working out in super-equipped gyms—can rarely gain muscle at all?

I could give you lots of reasons. Routine in eating and working is one. The motivation to train hard is one more. Absence of distractions is yet another. But there's a bigger reason. I have been asked on many occasions if there's a natural alternative for steroids—and I always answer the same: there is, but you can't buy it from a drugstore. It's called *sleep*. During sleep, your brain essentially orders your body to produce its own performance-enhancing drugs.

Inmates sleep like *kings*. I'm not saying that shit's right, but there it is. Behind bars, when it's time for Lights Out, you go to sleep. The time is always the same in the same institution—regular as clockwork. This is, essentially, how our ancestors lived—the sun goes down (Lights Out) and the brain and nervous system switch off for a well-deserved supercharge. Many convicts get ten hours per night—often with daily naps thrown in for good measure.

On the outside, it's totally different. Folks can control their own artificial sunlight, using bulbs, lamps, LCD TVs, laptops and phones. They can go out and drink, or party, or watch Netflix all night, if they want. As a result, the sleeping patterns of most people today—especially young people—are *chaos*. And they wonder why they are plagued with insomnia and sleep problems...their brains don't have a f***in clue what's going on! There is no routine at all, and they definitely don't get enough sleep—the average modern American gets well under seven hours, often much less than that.

Many training writers lump "rest and sleep" together under the same category. This is a mistake. Sleep is

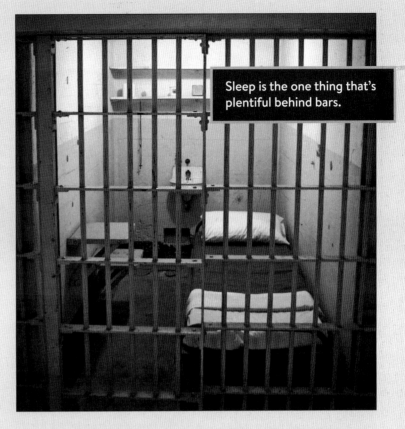

Sleep is the one thing that's plentiful behind bars.

a unique physiological condition. Ten minutes of sleep does not equate to ten minutes of rest...or twenty minutes of rest...or an hour of rest. Sleep does *everything* rest does for the body and brain, but the opposite ain't true. Don't get me wrong, I'm a big fan of programmed rest (see Commandment VI), but no amount of simple *rest* can give you what *sleep* is capable of. When you sleep:

- Your brain produces *Growth Hormone (GH)*—dangerous, expensive and illegal on the streets, but healthy and free if you take a nap.

- The brain generates *natural melatonin*—possibly the most powerful immunity and healing compound known to science. (As well as helping muscles heal, high melatonin levels may even ward off cancer. This stuff is magic!)

- When you sleep, your brain produces *Luteinizing Hormone (LH)*, which (in dudes) strongly stimulates the interstitial cells of your *cojones* to produce testosterone—the number-one bodybuilding chemical powerhouse.

And that's just a taster of what sleep does for a bodybuilder. Sleep is the cornerstone of muscle growth—and if that doesn't persuade you to try and get more sleep at night (daily naps are great, too), then how about this: *extra sleep can make you ripped.*

It's not something most people understand, but your sleep-wake cycles even regulate your eating patterns. Back when our species was evolving, the annual fruiting season occurred during late summer—when the days were at their *longest*. During this time, our ancestors went crazy trying to gobble up all the carb-heavy fruit they could find, to build thick bodyfat stores to protect us from the harsh, hungry winter round the corner.

These days, most everyone (outside jails) artificially prolongs their daylight time to ridiculous lengths using the bright electric lights in their home, not to mention the flickering boob tube, video games, etc. As a result, their Paleolithic brains still think they're stuck in late summer—*all year round*. So they react accordingly, continually pumping out neurotransmitters and hormones programmed to make them guzzle down all the carbs we can find. No wonder folks can't stick to diets. Their brains are trying to make them eat to survive winter!

Get to bed early, and your internal calendar won't be tricked into thinking it's fruiting season—you'll find you're suddenly not craving carbs like a maniac. It works.

Sleep also causes your fat cells to express *leptin*—sometimes called the "lean hormone". Leptin regulates bodyfat expenditure and sparks up the release of energy from your fatty tissue. Go have a nap before you read the next Commandment, Jack. You might have a six-pack when you wake up.

If you want to build mass and blow-torch your bodyfat like Danny Kavadlo, skip the supplements and focus on getting more sleep!

COMMANDMENT IX: TRAIN THE MIND ALONG WITH THE BODY!

This is a truism. The role of *the mind* in training is so fundamental that many books fail to even discuss it. The bodybuilders of the classical era sure understood it however, and they understood it well. Vince Gironda—"Iron Guru" and the *real* "Trainer of Champions", including first Mr Olympia, Larry Scott—was once asked what he thought was the ultimate supplement. This was his answer:

The Iron Guru bent a few pullup bars, That's for sure.

"...no supplement company has come up with a pill or powder as powerful as the mind. Conversely, the mind can equal and surpass any food supplement...if that is what you want from the mind.

Those weights never did anything for me. They never whispered in my ear. They never said, "curl me. Do this four times, or that for so many weeks." I can dictate to the weights. I can dictate to my body. OK? Do I need to say any more on that?"

— Larry Scott, The Wild Physique (Column), Musclemag no. 132

Isaac Newton taught us that an arrow will fly straight and true forever—unless external forces (like friction, gravity, etc.) drag it to a standstill. I strongly believe that the human mind is like this. It goes in the right direction just fine—*until negative influences drag it down*. These negative influences are destructive ideas and damaging thought-patterns. As far as bodyweight training goes, there are *six* major classes of these ideas which screw with our training—or make us quit altogether.

Combating and defeating these six groups of negative ideas—I call them *training* demons—is at the heart of successful training. The topic is too deep to discuss here, but those of you who are interested can find more in chapter 21 of **Convict Conditioning 2**—*The Mind: Escaping the True Prison*.

COMMANDMENT X: GET STRONG!

If you want a quick summary of this article, it's this: *strength* is built quickest by training the *nervous system*. *Mass* is built quickest by training the *muscles*. Over the last 9 Commandments, I've shown you the best, most powerful strategies you can use to train your muscles.

Does that mean that I'm telling you to permanently steer clear of strength training, if your only goal is to get bigger? *No*—and here's why.

The relationship between the nervous system and the muscular system is a bit like the relation between an *electrical circuit* (the nervous system) and a *light bulb* (the muscles). The higher you turn the wattage on the circuit, the brighter the bulb will glow. Likewise, the higher you amp up the nervous system (through *improved motor unit recruitment* and *neural facilitation*), the harder your muscles will contract and the stronger you are.

A bodybuilder primarily trains his (or her) *muscles* —they are constantly buying bigger light bulbs. A pure strength athlete primarily trains his (or her) *nervous system*—they keep their small light bulb, and simply turn up the wattage on the circuit. You can have very powerful bulbs that are only tiny, just as there exist superhumanly strong athletes with relatively small muscles.

The electric light analogy: think of the bulb as your muscle mass, the wattage as your nervous power.

Here's the thing—from a certain point of view, both these athletes want the same thing; more "light", which, in our analogy, means more *work output* from the muscles. Athletes who truly want maximum *strength* also train their muscles—they buy bigger bulbs. You see this in powerlifting, weightlifting and similar strength events; as athletes grow in strength, they also increase in mass, often competing in several higher weight classes through their careers. A strong, big athlete is always stronger than a strong, small one.

From the opposite end, bodybuilders want more "light" (more capacity for muscular work output) because it allows them to use harder exercises and lift more, to direct a greater stimulus to their *muscles* for greater adaptation—higher and higher levels of mass gains. Everyone understands this—the larger and larger a bodybuilder becomes, the greater the weight they have to lift to retain their gains and keep making progress.

In other words; if you wish to gain as much muscle as your genetic potential will allow, just training your *muscles* won't cut it. You need to train your *nervous system* too—at least some of the time.

Have you ever noticed that guys who begin bodybuilding make progress and build size for 3-6 months, then it grinds to a halt? This is why. They have literally *run out of strength*. How hard you can train your muscles—how much stress you can put them through—partially depends on how strong you are. If that novice then committed 3-6 months to training their *nervous systems* instead of their *muscles* and building up their pure strength, they would find they could subsequently return to their bodybuilding-style training, and they'd experience another big spurt of growth.

Classic bodybuilders all understood this relationship between size and strength. Many of them devoted 3-6 months per year working full bore to train their nervous system, to get as insanely strong as they could, unworried about their muscle size during that time. Others performed pure strength work *alongside* their bodybuilding, either during different sessions or mixed and matched. Successful bodybuilders today do the same—they mix "hypertrophy" (growth) work with "strength" work. They understand that just one won't work too well without the other.

Joe Greenstein—"The Mighty Atom"—weighed 140lbs, soaking wet. But he was so damn strong he could change a tire on a car, without using a jack! He could break three rounds of steel chain wrapped around his ribs, just through lung expansion. He bent steel bars and drove thick nails through pine using one hand wrapped in thin cloth (above). If big muscles and big strength were the same, this would be impossible. His light bulbs were tiny, but damn—his wattage was turned up to the max!

The take-home message of this? Simple. Muscular training is what builds size, but without added *strength* your progress only lasts so long. You'll get better gains if you cycle (or mix in) pure bodyweight strength training—where you train your nervous system—with your bodyweight bodybuilding.

The next question is—*how* do you train your nervous system for pure strength, using bodyweight techniques?

I got ya covered chief. I included a special strength-without-size tutorial with all the strategies you need for jacking up that electrical circuit! Check out chapter six: *The Democratic Alternative…how to get as powerful as possible without gaining a pound.*

To recap, here are the Ten C-MASS Commandments, all in one shot:

THE 10 COMMANDMENTS OF CALISTHENICS MASS

I: Embrace Reps!

II: Work Hard!

III: Use Simple, Compound Exercises!

IV: Limit Sets!

V: Focus on Progress—and Utilize a Training Journal!

VI: You Grow When You Rest. So Rest!

VII: Quit Eating "Clean" the Whole Time!

VIII: Sleep More!

IX: Train the Mind Along With the Body!

X: Get Strong!

I don't envy bodybuilding newbies today. There is information overload like never before! If you are barraged by a huge amount of contradictory information in the magazines, on TV, from your friends and on the internet, trying to find a coherent bodybuilding philosophy that works can be murder.

These ten rules are simple. If every bodybuilder followed them, there would be *tons* more muscle in America in just a few weeks.

3

"Coach" Wade's Bodypart Tactics

O kay, bro. We've chatted about the *theory* of bodyweight muscle gain—now let's get down and dirty and talk *tools*. Anybody who picks up a muscle rag knows which machine or dumbbell exercise works their pecs and lats or whatever, but those bodybuilders deciding to take calisthenics seriously might not know what their options are. I got you covered, sonny. In this section we're gonna look at techniques for 11 major body areas.

Pure bodyweight, boy. No excuses.

QUADZILLA! (...AND QUADZOOKIE.)

The Gold Standard quad developer is squatting—and the Big Daddy is the *one-legged squat*, all the way down (slow, Jack) until the calves and hammies are compressed together. Then push the piston back up: no bouncing, no rocking. Your basic bodyweight work should be built around progressions to get you to this exercise.

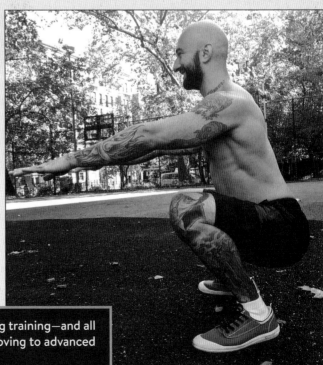

The bodyweight squat is the foundation of all leg training—and all human movement. Perfect the basics before moving to advanced variations, such as one-leg "pistols".

Al Kavadlo is a great proponent of the shrimp squat as a basic leg press-style bodyweight movement. These are performed by holding the heel of one leg to your ass, while you squat down until the knee of the same leg touches the ground. Al makes this exercise look easy—it isn't. It's a wonderful quad and glute builder, and is certainly comparable to the one-leg squat in terms of difficulty. Advanced athletes can increase difficulty by standing on a base—this radically increases the range-of-motion. Al calls these *jumbo* shrimp squats! (Pretty sure he invented the name.) Just as tasty, but with added muscle.

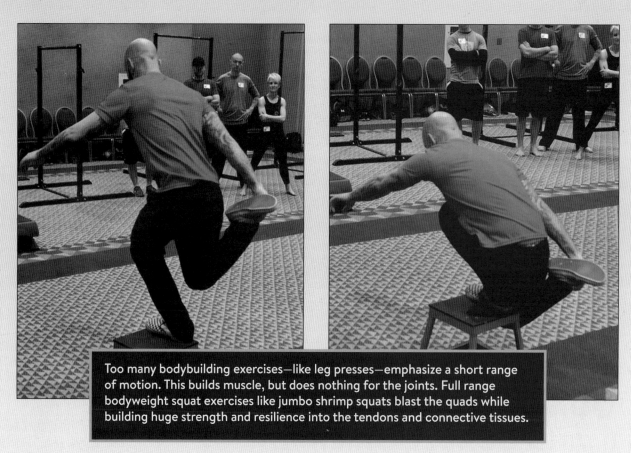

Too many bodybuilding exercises—like leg presses—emphasize a short range of motion. This builds muscle, but does nothing for the joints. Full range bodyweight squat exercises like jumbo shrimp squats blast the quads while building huge strength and resilience into the tendons and connective tissues.

Other valuable basics are typically based on the way the legs were built to move—explosive jumping is a great example. Jumps not only build power, speed and tendon strength, but they also carry-over real well into your squats. What is a vertical jump, if not a real fast squat? How about:

- Box jumps
- Tuck jumps
- One-leg jumps, etc.
- Vertical jump
- Split jumps
- Dead leaps
- Long jumps

All jumps also work the calves, glutes, hamstrings and waist—in fact, explosive jumps should be total-body moves: bring those arms along for the ride. For all explosive work, keep your reps low (1-3) and sets moderate (around 5) to maintain that crisp, fresh spring in your technique. (*Convict Conditioning 3*, the next volume in the series, is gonna be a complete textbook of progressive explosive calisthenics. It'll be invaluable to fighters, football players, and pretty much all serious athletes. Keep an eye out for that sucker, huh?)

Are these basics—one-leg squats and explosive work—enough to give you great quads? Hell yes! Build to two sets of twenty *deep* one-leg squats per leg, and follow that with a five sets of vertical jumps, where you beat 25 inches on your top set.* Then you'll agree with me. If anyone you meet tells you that bodywork won't build strong, functional legs, challenge them to do the same—and enjoy a good laugh as the f***ers *fail*.

In-gym bodybuilders love to isolate their quads with ligament-wrecking machine exercises like leg extensions. There are superior bodyweight alternatives—enter the *sissy squat*.

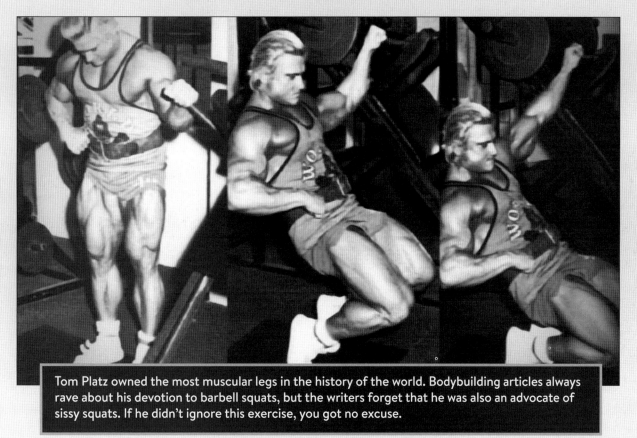

Tom Platz owned the most muscular legs in the history of the world. Bodybuilding articles always rave about his devotion to barbell squats, but the writers forget that he was also an advocate of sissy squats. If he didn't ignore this exercise, you got no excuse.

A genuine sissy squat is pretty hard to describe—I'll do my best, but you're probably well-advised to find one of the many videos on the web. (If you search, be aware that some gyms have sissy squat stations, but ironically it is impossible to perform a kosher sissy squat when using one of these death-traps. Avoid.) A description: grab a sturdy object for balance, and get up on tippy-toes. Bend the knees but without bending at the hips; this will mean that you start leaning back as your knees dip forwards, angling towards the ground. Some athletes have such strong tendons that their knees touch the ground! Finish a leg workout with two sets of 20 sissys and your quads will shape up in a hurry. Not my favorite exercise, but many old timers swore by them, performed along with deep-knee bends. The Iron Guru, Vince Gironda—great bodybuilding ideologist of the Golden Era, and trainer of a young Mr. Schwarzenegger—also swore by sissy squats. He wouldn't let anyone perform barbell squats in his gym!

*A true vertical jump is measured from *above* your top reach, not from *under* your feet. If you don't know how to perform a vertical jump, Google *Sargent Vertical Jump Test*.

Why are they called "sissy squats"? Two theories. One is that they are named in honor of the mythological King Sisyphus, who was condemned to roll a boulder uphill every day in the afterlife, only to watch it roll back down at midnight. (I guess the sissy squat position does look a little like you are pushing back against something; like pushing a car uphill with your back to it.) The less literary etymology—and probably the correct one—is that the exercise places the quads in such an isolated position that the technique is incredibly hard to do, turning even a big strong man into a "sissy".

HAMSTRINGS: STAND SIDEWAYS WITH PRIDE

You can't work hamstrings with bodyweight—I've heard this kind of shit for years, by folks who simply don't know any better. Truth be told, I've seen a number of calisthenics athletes with awesome back-legs. It makes sense if you think about it; the human body evolved *millions* of years before barbells were invented…why do you think God put 'em back there, if they had nothing to do?! So sure you can work your hammies with calisthenics.

For a start, one of the main roles of the hamstrings is to assist the quadriceps during squatting motions. Typically, antagonistic muscles like these are not supposed to fire at the same time while a limb is moving, but the hamstrings and quads work *together* during squats—big time! This apparent breech in the laws of kinesiology is called *Lombard's Paradox*, and it means that if you are already performing bodyweight squats of some kind, you are working your hamstrings! You… you *are* squatting, right?

As well as bodyweight squat progressions, the other basic exercise you should be performing for the hamstrings is *bridging*. I've already said that bridging is the most important strength exercise in the world. Bridging works the entire posterior chain of muscles, and this includes the hamstrings, which work at the hips to press the torso back, and at the knees to keep the leg bent under load. You often see bridgers rising up onto their toes—this is a mistake. As a general rule of thumb, the quadriceps are activated by pressure through the *toes*—the hamstrings are activated by pressure through the *heels*. To work your hamstrings and activate your entire posterior chain, always push from your heels when you *are* bridging.

Of course, bridging is not a single movement but a family of movements. A form of *bridging* which is particularly stimulating to the hamstrings (not to mention the triceps!) is the *straight bridge*. If anybody has trouble building their hamstrings, I advise four/five sets of twenty slow, strict reps of straight bridges, followed by a series of sprints, or (better) hill sprints. That kind of shit would put muscle on a pencil.

Your hamstrings—*biceps femoris* for you smartasses—are part of your *posterior chain* of muscles. They are a two-part muscle (the "bi" in *biceps femoris*). One part is shorter, and only crosses the knee; this part helps bend the leg at the knee. The other part is pretty long and crosses the knee and hips and works with the glutes in pushing the trunk upwards and backwards. (This section of

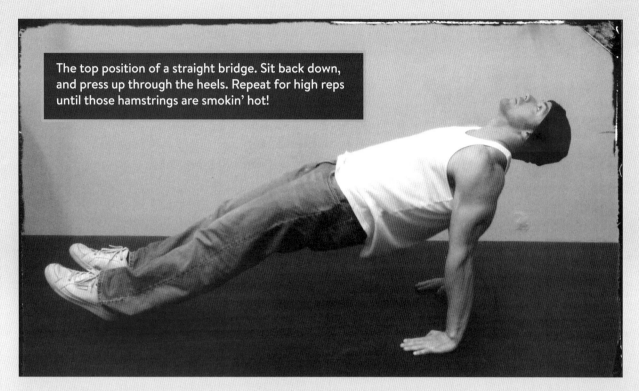

The top position of a straight bridge. Sit back down, and press up through the heels. Repeat for high reps until those hamstrings are smokin' hot!

the hamstring is so strong and long, that when Medieval butchers had to display hog legs, they would string them to the wall using the tendon of this muscle. That's where we get the word "hamstring". Ten bucks to you if you already knew that. Write me for your prize, but don't forget the twenty bucks postage, 'kay?)

The upshot of this is that the best way to isolate the hamstrings is to bend the knees against force—the kind of activity you see on a leg curl machine. Bodyweight training has its own variation of this exercise: the *bridge curl*. Lie supine (on ya back, dummy) with your heels up on a higher base—say the arm of a couch. Using pure hamstring power, push down through the heels as you bend the legs and lever yourself up onto your shoulders. This can be made progressive by the height of the base, strictness of form, and of course you can perform bridge curls unilaterally.

As with quads, explosive work is also essential for fully developed hamstrings. The legs were designed to work this way. What jumping is to the quads, sprinting is to the hamstrings. The hamstrings are worked very powerfully during sprints—which is why so many sprinters injure their hamstrings when they haven't warmed up correctly. The angle of incline is also a feature of interest for bodybuilders—the higher the incline, the harder the hamstrings have to work. Stair sprints are superior to regular sprints for building hammies, but hill sprints are best of all.

If you think these exercises are useless for bodybuilders, you've never looked at a goddam sprinter's legs, have ya? Not only do these exercises build muscle, they also build speed and strength, through ramping up the neural connections between the legs and brain. You want to look like a sprinter not a marathon runner though, so keep distances short (100 meters or under) and intense as hell. Any more than four of five runs is probably a waste of time, as your explosiveness will be spent by then.

SOFTBALL BICEPS

The best biceps exercise in the world is the *underhand pullup*—often just called the *chin-up*. This is *bar none*. Talk to most bodybuilders about biceps, and all they can shoot back is "barbell curls". Well, any muscle-builder worth his salt will tell ya that compound, multi-joint exercises are best for growth, because they allow you to overload the muscles better. But barbell curls are, in fact, an *isolation* exercise...it doesn't matter how much weight you use, you are still essentially moving at only *one* joint, the elbow joint. Pullups move joints at the elbow *and* the shoulder, making them a *true* compound exercise.

That matter of *overload*—the amount of force you are working with—is another issue. The neophyte 200lbs bodybuilder might be rocking 100lbs on barbell curls, but when he does his pullups, he's forcing those same biceps to shift *twice as much* weight. Just imagine how strong your biceps are by the time you can do one-arm pullups! Does that equate to greater size? Well, check out the Olympics; male gymnasts typically have better biceps than the weight-lifters!

So those of you looking for biceps exercises who aren't performing pullups regularly are really, *really* putting the cart before the horse. Make use of pullups *first*. When regular overhand pullups stop stimulating those biceps as much, you can add sets with the underhand grip—much more effective for the bis. To add progression, bring the hands closer over time. Once your grip is close and underhand-style, you have a serious biceps exercise in your bodyweight armory.

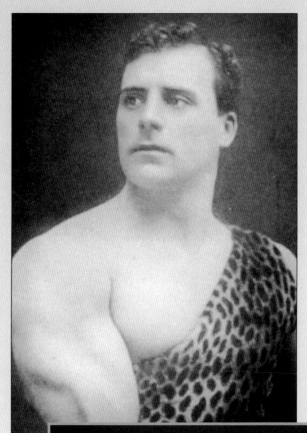

Scotsman William Bankier had the largest arms in the world before steroids were invented. He built his biceps exclusively using bodyweight movements.

You can still go further though—use the principles in **Convict Conditioning** or **Raising the Bar** to build to a one-arm underhand pullup. You can follow the same protocols with Australian pullups if you want, to hit your shit from a slightly different angle. Beats dumbbell curls anyday, kid.

Another great compound move for the biceps (and forearms) is *rope climbing*. As with all bodyweight, this can be performed progressively. At first, use your arms and legs; then use your arms and legs to climb, but descend with only your arms; finally, climb using just the arms. The old school strongmen often used to climb from sitting—and retain an L-hold position. This is arguably the Master Step of the rope climbing family. But there are alternatives. William Bankier "the

Scottish Hercules" built the world's biggest biceps back in the 19th Century, using nothing but rope climbing. He did utilize a brutally advanced variation, though; he would hitch up a rope diagonally (45 degrees) and climb it *backwards*, using pure arm power. Try that if you think you have strong guns. Rope climbing is a true discipline to itself in bodyweight training, and deserves more respect than it gets. I discuss rope work in **Convict Conditioning 2**. I also wrote more about it in my article *The Dirty Dozen* which my buddy Rob Drucker published on his cool old-school site *MusclesOfIron.com*.

Despite what some trainers may tell you, you can also perform bodyweight biceps *isolation* exercises—such as the classic (but-rarely-seen-in-gyms) *curl-up*. In order to stop your shoulders (read: *lats*) helping out as much with pullups, you can attach a plank over the front of your pullup unit, at the point where your forearms/elbows are located. (You can pad the plank if you need to.) This set-up means that when you pull yourself up, the elbows (pushing on the plank) cannot move forwards, and the biceps are forced to lever you up. Pure power! If you can build one, this old school piece of kit will give you biceps straight from Hades.

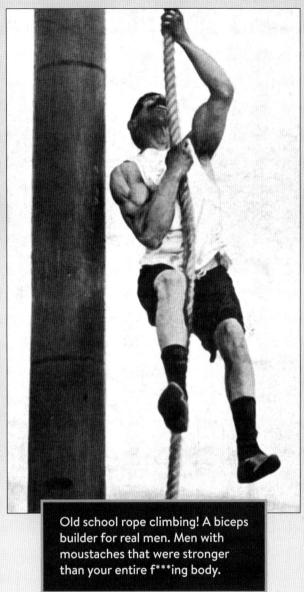

Old school rope climbing! A biceps builder for real men. Men with moustaches that were stronger than your entire f***ing body.

TITANIC TRICEPS

I tell you, I have *never* met a gym-trained bodybuilder who understands how the f***ing triceps really work. Not one. Occasionally you'll read an article by this or that "champ" saying that push-downs work the long head, or whatever, but these pricks typically contradict themselves because they are just going by what some clown in the gym told them. Google "triceps anatomy", and the majority of pics that come up will be totally wrong. Forget all that. I'm going to tell you right now how the triceps work. This stuff is gold—pay attention.

First up (and obviously) the triceps have three muscle heads. That's what "tri-ceps" means in Latin. ("Tri" is three, as in tri-angle; and "cep", or "cap" is head, as in *captain* or *decapitate*.) Let's look at 'em:

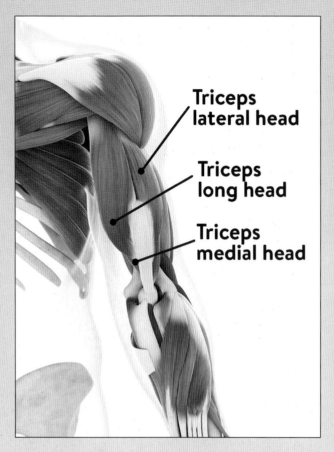

Triceps
lateral head

Triceps
long head

Triceps
medial head

The *lateral head* runs along the outside of the tris—this head is the outer crescent of the "horseshoe" in a well-built arm. Because this head doesn't cross the shoulder joint, it works as a powerful assistance muscle, straightening the arms when the big torso muscles are activated (particularly then the upper arm moves away from the torso while straightening). When the shoulder girdle and arm work in synergy to push, you have the classic pressing movements. E.g:

* All pushups
* Close pushups
* Handstand pushups
* Dips
* Bridges

The *long head* runs down the back of the tris—it's this largest head that hangs down under the arm like a shark's belly in a biceps pose. The long head crosses the shoulder as well as the elbow, so in addition to straightening the arm, it can also pull the upper arm *down*, towards the torso (as in a pullup. Yes, pullups work the triceps). It's a law of kinesiology that muscles which cross two joints work best at one end when the other end is *stretched*, so to work the long head via the elbow, your upper arms should be up and away from the torso, and remain as fixed as possible. For example:

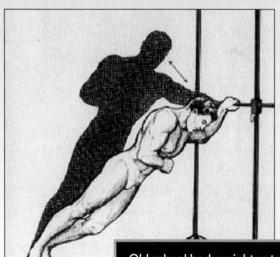

* Tiger bend pushups
* Tiger bend handstand pushups
* Bodyweight extensions

The *medial head* is on the inside of the tris—it's that stubby little lump next to the elbow. It's situated next to the elbow to give a little extra help with locking out the arms (although you don't need to lock the arm *perfectly* straight to activate this small muscle—a slight kink in your arms is in fact

Old school bodyweight extensions—the Master Step! You can make this triceps exercise easier by using two hands, varying your grip, changing bar height, kneeling or altering your waist angle.

best, because *completely* locking out tends to shift the load from your triceps onto your skeletal structure). The key to working this muscle then, is not so much in the exercise you use, but in the difficulty of that exercise. It you are struggling to push to a rep to lockout, you are working the medial head. So pick the big, tough presses like:

- Handstand pushups
- One-arm pushups
- Dips
- Straight bridges
- Korean dips

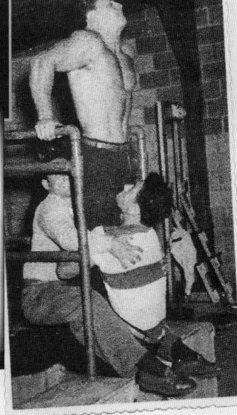

Bronx boy Marvin Eder was the world's greatest dipper. He performed dips with two guys hanging off his legs...for a total of 434 lbs. He didn't need isolation work!

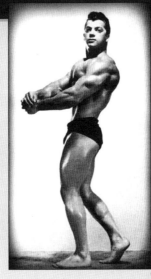

In reality, all these muscle-heads like to work as a *unit* if they can. To recruit them as a team, you need the challenge of a heavy load. This equals lots of hard presses, using the most bodyweight you can—one-arm pushups, handstand pushups, and dips are the "Big Three" here. Work these hard, and you are unlikely to need anything else. Certainly the usual pansy-pant bodybuilding advice of cable exercises and kickbacks are a waste of time if you want to really build your triceps. Hit 'em heavy with HARD exercises, or go home!

Those of you who want a little extra arm work (beyond the "Big Three") should throw in one of the specialist *long head* movements listed above. More than this is unnecessary. Triceps get a lot of work in a well-structured bodyweight routine—even ab work like the L-hold can hit the triceps hard—so don't overdo it like so many body-builders do. Stick to the basics and only add in more when you really have to.

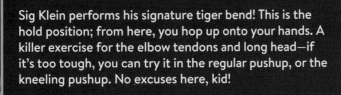

Sig Klein performs his signature tiger bend! This is the hold position; from here, you hop up onto your hands. A killer exercise for the elbow tendons and long head—if it's too tough, you can try it in the regular pushup, or the kneeling pushup. No excuses here, kid!

FARMER FOREARMS

I wrote what I consider the definitive mini-manual of calisthenics forearm and grip training in my book *Convict Conditioning 2*. I can't recount all that here, but the take-home message is that the forearms are best built through gripping exercises, and you can build superhuman grip by utilizing intelligent hanging progressions. Hanging beats those crush-style grippers that are so popular because it trains all the fingers (and thumbs!) equally and does not involve *torque*, which grippers demand, and which destroys the knuckles and fingers of so many unwary athletes.

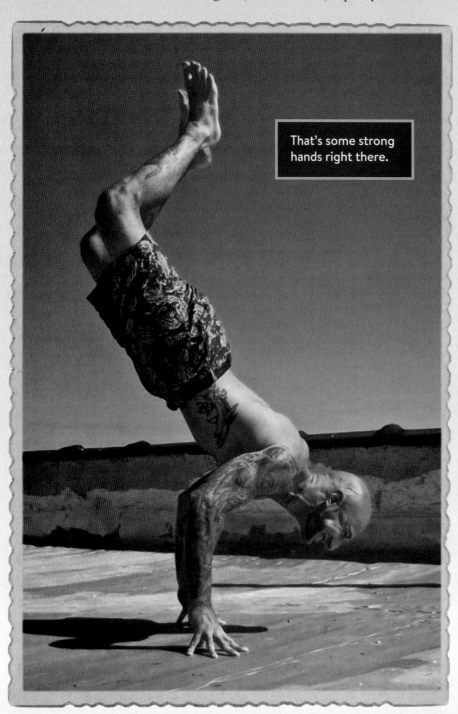

That's some strong hands right there.

Hangs should be balanced out with fingertip pushups for the top side of the forearms and hands—again, don't just rush into fingertip pushups if you ain't used to it; you can damage those delicate digits. Instead, use a loving, progressive course of exercises, like the one I set out for ya. Your fingers will thank you bro.

In addition to the big basics, bodyweight offers a large number of *isometric* kung fu-style hand and grip exercises. Bear in mind that *any* hand/finger movement, performed slowly and with "dynamic tension" will add power to the deep tissues of the hands and forearms. Many of these are excellent for building tendon strength. This is a fun journey, kiddo. Experiment.

IT'S NOT "ABS" IT'S "MIDSECTION", BITCH

Right, every shitty fitness website has a dozen articles on "abs" and every muscle rag on the newsstand is (every f***ing week!) a "special" on abs. So in order to separate myself from this garbage, I'm going to keep my abs advice as short and sharp as possible.

Avoid modern views on abs at all costs. If a magazine says something, you would be well advised to promptly do the f***ing opposite. If some no-dick personal trainer tells you to do your ab movements on an inflated Swiss ball, drop to the concrete instead. If they tell you to forget counting reps and try to *feel* your abs tensing and burning, instantly forget how your abs feel and focus on *counting reps* instead. If they tell you to go with short-stroke isolation movements, immediately start performing the biggest moves you can find. Capiche?

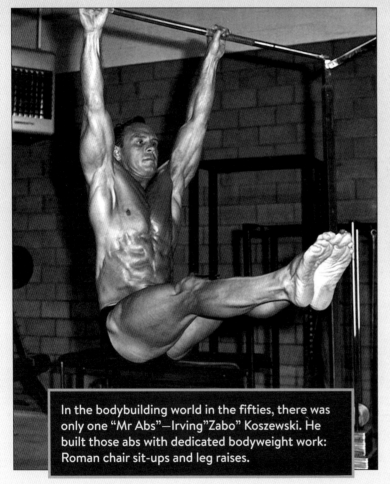

In the bodybuilding world in the fifties, there was only one "Mr Abs"—Irving"Zabo" Koszewski. He built those abs with dedicated bodyweight work: Roman chair sit-ups and leg raises.

Don't become one of those pricks who sees midsection work ("abs") as a light, ancillary exercise, sometimes done half-heartedly for a few sets at the end of a workout. At the other end of the spectrum, *don't* become one of those phaggots who sees "core" exercises as the be-all end-all of training, who ploughs through fifty weak-ass movements five times per week.

As a bodybuilder, your method should be to pick a big, tough midsection movement and work at it hard and progressively to thicken your six-pack. This work should be a cornerstone of your training, no different from pullups or squats. It's a requirement.

Which movements to pick? Sit-ups are okay, but leg raises are better—particularly if they are done hanging from an overhead bar. Leg raises aren't just one movement, remember—the *PCC Instructor's Manual* illustrates eleven progressively more difficult leg raises, and details over forty variations in the leg raise "family" (not counting static midsection holds, which are detailed in a later chapter). Leg raises are a compound exercise. They work the *abdominals*, but also the crucial (to combat, running, etc.) *hip flexors*, and the deep muscles of the thighs (*rectus femoris*). The hanging position forces the entire anterior chain to work as a family, including the grip and arms, the *lats, serratus* and *intercostals* of the ribcage. This "chain" was built to work together.

Always avoid "isolation" exercises like crunches; they are designed to strengthen only one area of the chain. What would happen in real life if an engineer tried to use a chain with only ONE strong link? You got it, the f***ing thing would break, right?! And that's just what happens to men who exclusively do the typical isolation-only ab routines. Something breaks. They always have a bad back, a hernia, rib pain, a bad knee, or what have you. So train your midsection with big, compound exercises! In the words of the late, great Alan Calvert:

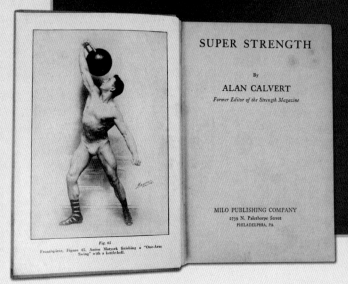

"It is possible to develop the abdominal muscles in a certain way without bringing out much development in the front of the thigh. In my opinion, this is a foolish way to develop any set of muscles. Muscles are not just for appearance, but for use; and if your front thighs and abdominal muscles are developed in concert, they will be much better developed and very much stronger than if you attempt to develop the abdominal muscles alone."

— Alan Calvert, Super Strength (1924)

SUPER STRENGTH

By

ALAN CALVERT

Former Editor of the Strength Magazine

MILO PUBLISHING COMPANY
2739 N. Palethorpe Street
PHILADELPHIA, PA.

Fig. 65
Frontispiece, Figure 65. Anton Matysek finishing a "One-Arm Swing" with a kettle-bell.

The old timers knew their shit, right? As I've said, I would steer clear of most modern advice on midsection work. But if you really want to become a Master of the Midsection, there is only one manual I recommend on gut training: **Diamond-Cut Abs** by Danny Kavadlo. That book is the *ultimate* advanced textbook on everything to do with waist training, and should belong in the library of all serious athletes. If you know about Danny, you know he is a calisthenics master in the old school style. His coaching is simple, healthy and productive, and if you've ever seen the guy's abs it's clear that this approach works better than the rest!

A final tip, kid. Your abdominal muscles consist of more than the "six pack" (the *abdominis rectus*). This is only the *outer* layer of muscle. There are three basic layers in the gut: first you have the outer abdominals, followed by the *oblique* muscles, followed by the *transversus* muscle layer. Leg raises will work the outer layer perfectly. The obliques should be worked by side-to-side and rotational movements: I recommend that if you are going to work these areas, follow the same "compound" approach as for working your six-pack and systematically train them as part of your entire "lateral chain". As ever, avoid machines, gizmos and informercial gadgets. You need twists and flags. For full zero-to-hero progressions on the twist and flag, check *Convict Conditioning 2.*

The deepest layer, the transversus, keeps the stomach pulled in. (you know how you pulled your gut in, last time a hot chick walked into the room? That was your little buddy the transversus doing that for ya.) This layer is crucial to strength and health, because every time we make an effort—like picking up a fridge—the diaphragm contracts and intra-abdominal pressure skyrockets as a result. If the transversus isn't fit and strong enough to contain this belly pressure it can split, allowing a piece of intestine to bulge out. This is called a hernia. So don't ignore your transversus. The simplest way to train your transversus is to consciously keep your stomach *tensed* and *drawn in tight* during every single rep of midsection work: this is the method I advise in *Convict Conditioning.* But if you want to get more serious about training your transversus (as well as your intercostals, diaphragm, and all the muscles involved in respiration), you need to explore the old school art and science of *deep breathing.* I'll talk more about this under chest training, which is up next.

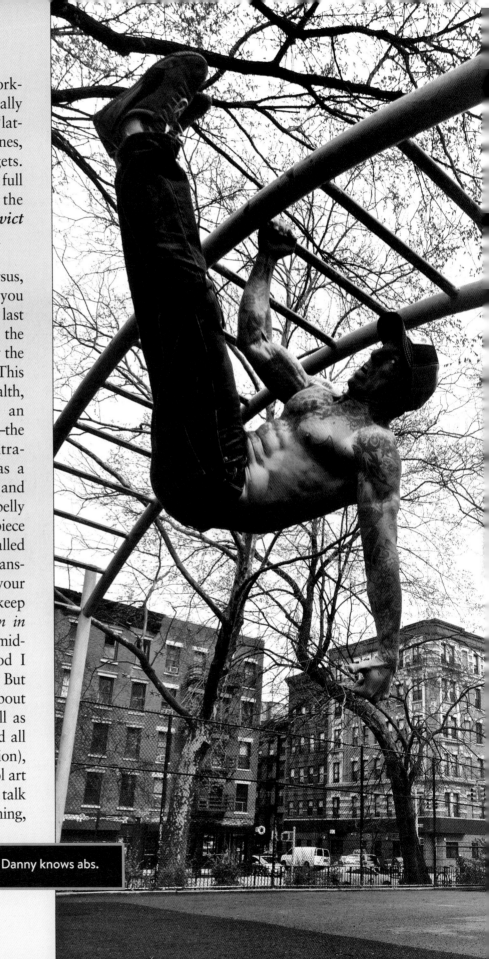

Danny knows abs.

MAXIMUM CHEST

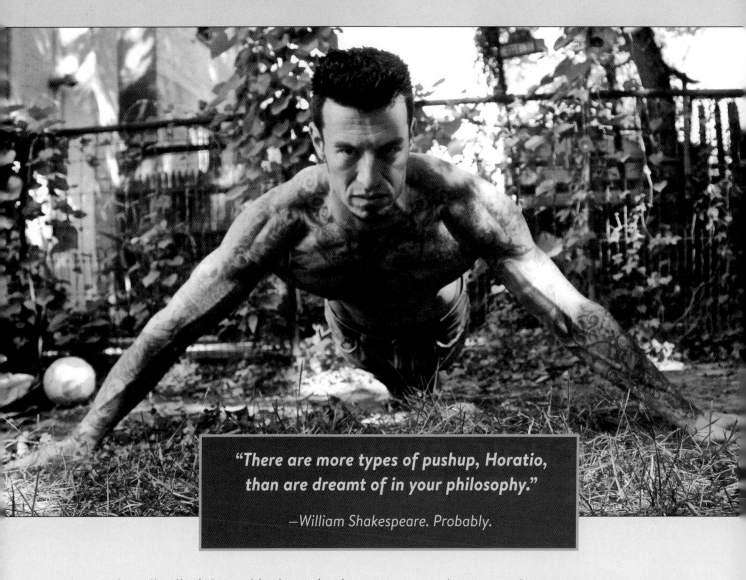

*"There are more types of pushup, Horatio,
than are dreamt of in your philosophy."*

—William Shakespeare. Probably.

The roll call of classical bodyweight chest exercises is dynamic and impressive. It's an ancient, effective, tactical buffet of super-moves, brother. You know I'm talkin' bout the *pushup* family, right? *Pushups* and *pecs* go together like booze and strippers, son! I'm talking:

- Incline pushups
- Decline pushups
- Classic pushups
- Stretch pushups between chairs
- Jackknife pushups
- Cat stretch pushups
- Divebomber pushups
- Hindu pushups

- Maltese pushups
- Ring pushups
- Asymmetrical pushups
- Snake pushups
- Archer pushups
- Tripod pushups
- Prison pushups
- …and dozens more!

If you are working with any of these beauties you are training your pecs. These are all compound exercises, and they are better for it; sure, calisthenics pec isolation exercises are possible—such as bodyweight "flyes" using gymnastic rings—but frankly the chest muscles are built so fast with proper progressive bodyweight presses, there's usually no need for such shenanigans.

I typically advise a chest routine solidly founded on progressive *pushups*. Most dedicated bodyweight athletes thrive on pushups, but occasionally I get a guy with such sturdy arms and shoulders that they get the lion's share of the load during pushups. When this happens, their arms become more and more powerful, until ultimately the pecs barely get a look in when he does pressing movements. From that point on, it can become very hard to build pecs, because whatever the athlete tries the triceps take over and handle the load, like overprotective poppas.

What should you do if this is you? Focus on *dipping progressions*. I definitely favor pushups, because they are much less stressful on the

First Mr Olympia, Larry Scott, works some ring flyes for the pecs.

shoulders, elbows and forearms, for reasons I've discussed elsewhere. But—if you can adapt to it—there's no doubt that dipping has something special to offer bodybuilders. Why? Well, if you could cut open pecs and check out the direction of the deepest muscle fibers, you'd notice something weird—that most of them are angled more *downwards* than *outwards*. The upshot of this is that the pecs are much, much better at pushing *down* that *forwards*.

This might seem kinda strange, since most chest training is based on pushing *out*, away from the body—like in a pushup, or a bench press. But if you take a moment to think about it, it's true; the average *reasonably fit* 180lbs male could probably do several bodyweight dips, even if they hadn't really trained for it. But they are very, very unlikely to be able to perform a 180lbs bench press first time of asking, right? This is because the pecs are stronger at pushing *down* than *out* (it's also because the lats can support the shoulder girdle real well when pushing down, but that's another story.)

This is a major reason why *dippers* tend to have better pecs than pushup guys. Look at Al Kavadlo as an example. He has a lean, athletic physique, because he trains for that look. But his pecs are thick as a bodybuilder's—they stand out thick and deep, from his collarbones to his sternum.

Is it a coincidence that Al's favorite exercise is the muscle-up? (He's known as the *Monarch of Muscle-Ups* at the Dragon Door offices for a reason!) And what's a muscle-up if it's not a pullup with a straight-bar dip at the end? Guys like myself—who focused much more on flat pushups—wound up with thick triceps and forearms, and very powerful front delts, but without the stand-out huge pecs of the dip guys.

If you are serious about dipping for pec development, then your ultimate goal should be mastering dips on a straight horizontal bar—like at the top of a muscle-up, but without dropping all the way down, under the bar. In the PCC this is called a *horizontal bar dip*. Regular dipping involves pushing off parallel bars; these allow you to place your hands to your side. The side-on hand position allows the powerful lats to assist in the dip push (some athletes get sorer lats than pecs when they dip). However the more advanced *horizontal bar dip* involves the athlete pushing up with the hands forced *in front* of the bar; and when your hands are in front of you, the lats are "disabled" and less able

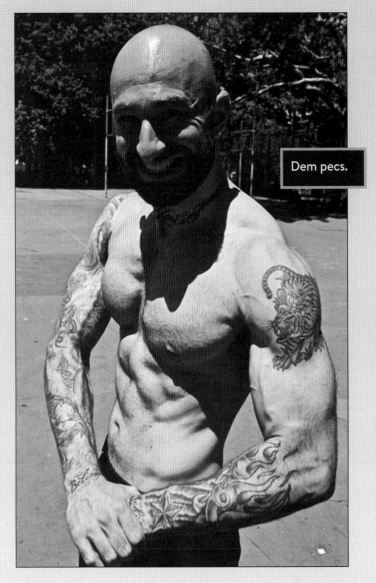

Dem pecs.

to help—so the majority of the workload is shifted onto the pecs. I have never seen an athlete who can handle double figures in the horizontal bar dip who doesn't have thick, imposing pectoral muscles. If you need it, it WILL do the same for you.

A couple final thoughts on chest training. Remember that your chest is composed of various muscles. Bodybuilders often talk "pecs", but as well as the large *pectoralis major*—which brings the arms in towards the torso—you also possess a pair of smaller *pectoralis minor* muscles—which help pull the shoulder socket *down* and *forward*. The pec minor gives much-neded depth to the upper chest and should not be ignored by bodybuilders.

You can work your pec minor with downwards presses such as dips and incline pushups, but I'm convinced that the finest exercise for these muscles isn't a press at all—it's *hanging*. If you are hanging with the shoulders nice and "tight" (i.e., pulled down, not left loose and stretched), then the pec minor is fulfilling its special stabilizing function, and will get thicker and stronger as a

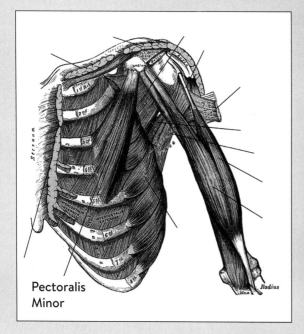

Pectoralis
Minor

result. So as well as working your back, lats, biceps, abs and triceps, pullups also work your freakin' pecs! Any hang will work though—hanging leg raises, monkey bar work, side-swings, hang grips. Whatever your flavor, man.

What we call a chest is about more than the pectorals, whether major or minor. If you think about it, a "big" chest also means a boxy, athletic ribcage. The ribcage is attached to lungs which can be trained to make it expand further, become larger—the rib muscles (*intercostals*), *serratus*, and the *diaphragm* which inflates the lungs. If there is a

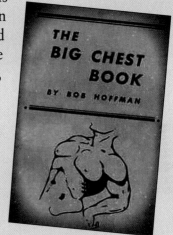

major difference between old school (pre-sixties) chest training and modern methods, it's this: the old timers used to train the *ribcage* as well as the external showy muscles which hang off it. How? Deep breathing exercises. These guys had such powerful chests and lungs that they could balloon their chests strongly enough to break chains wrapped around their bodies; they could explode hot water bottles by blowing into them; they could lie under boards and have vehicles driven over their torsos; and they sure as hell never ran out of breath when they did their bodyweight squats! From Sandow onwards, every strongman worth his salt a hundred years ago had his own method, his own system of deep breathing. These systems still exist in their manuals, if you search for them. (A good distillation of the old school attitude to chest training can be found in Bob Hoffman's 1950s work: *The Big Chest Book*. It's published free on the wonderful *Sandowplus* website, so Google it and read it.)

Pierre Gasnier could break chains wrapped around his chest—just like Superman.

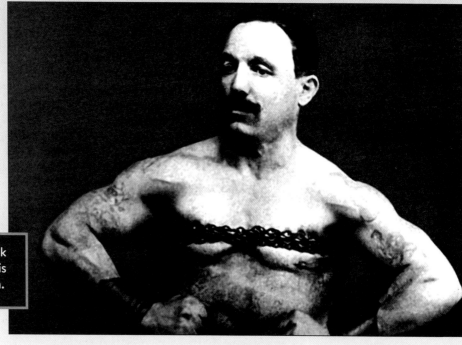

POWERFUL, HEALTHY SHOULDERS

The round, brawny cap of muscular armor covering the top of your shoulder is called a *deltoid*. The muscle was named by classically educated Renaissance anatomists, who decided that it looks kinda like the Greek letter *delta*. Smartasses.

Delta

All die-hard bodybuilders need to know is that the deltoids have three heads. One at the front (the *anterior deltoid*), one at the side (the *lateral*, or *medial deltoid*), and one at the back (the *posterior deltoid*). All these heads work together somewhat, but different heads take over at different angles:

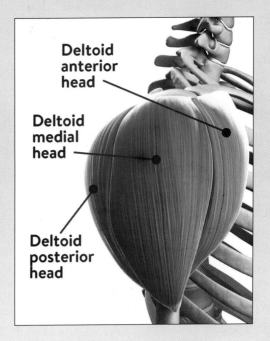

Deltoid anterior head

Deltoid medial head

Deltoid posterior head

- When you are moving your upper arms *forwards* (think: pushups, dips), you are working the front head;
- When you are moving your upper arms *upwards*, towards or past your head (think *handstands, handstand pushups, bridges*), you are working the side head;
- When you are moving your upper arms *backwards*, either towards the body or behind it (think *pullups, Aussie pullups*), you are working the rear head.

The first thing to notice here is that the deltoids actually get a lot of work from basic upper-body exercises. If you are doing pushups, handstand work and pullups, all three heads are getting worked.

If you want to give any of your shoulder heads an enhanced, specialist workout, a great tactic is to perform your basic exercises, but with a *wider* hand placement. As a rule of thumb, the closer your hand placement on an exercise, the more your *arms* take on the load; the further apart your hands, the more the *shoulder* heads do. Why? Because the torso muscles are attached high on your upper-arm bones, so they work better when the upper arms are close to the torso, such as you get with a medium-style hand placement—that's why most people are at their strongest with a shoulder-width grip on any given exercise. Closer than this and the torso muscles can't work real well, and the arms have to man up and do the work. At the other end of the spectrum, a wider-than-shoulder hand placement forces the elbows (and the humerus) out, away from the torso, and the torso muscles can't work very well there either, so the deltoid heads step in.

Take for example, classic pushups. A regular grip works the arms and front of the shoulders fairly equally; but as soon as you bring the hands close together, the movement turns into a monster of a triceps workout. Spread your hands as wide as you can, and the shoulders suddenly get worked harder (along with the chest muscles, which work in conjunction with the front delts). The same is true for handstand pushups; a close hand position is really a strength feat for the elbows and surrounding musculature; but use a wide hand position and the lateral deltoids will start screaming for mercy.

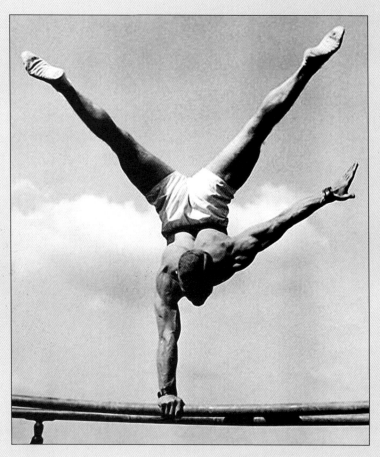

It's a myth that wide-grip pullups work the lats better than medium-grip; remember, a medium grip is best for torso muscles, like the lats. A wide grip works the (rear) shoulders. Close grip pullups are a go-to biceps exercise, but take a wide grip and suddenly your rear delts wake up and pop out to say hi. (For what it's worth, if you *really* want to build your rear delts, wide grip *horizontal pulls* should be your number one exercise. Your rear deltoids activate more strongly when pulling *backwards*—as with horizontal pulls—than *downwards*—as with pullups. As I mentioned before, this is because the deltoids work better when the elbows remain *out*, away from the body, and this occurs more with horizontal pulls than with pullups, where the elbows gradually head *towards* the body.)

This approach is the best way to perform specialist deltoid training; athletes really don't require isolation exercises. This is as true for regular weight-training as it is for bodyweight training. In order to express the forces of the torso in 360 degrees, the shoulder joint is incredibly versatile and mobile, but it pays for this mobility with a definite vulnerability. Moving away from natural, multi-joint movements and into the territory of artificial, isolation exercises can place angular strain on the shoulder joints which they never evolved to accommodate. The result is shoulder injury, rotator cuff tears, frozen shoulder and chronic pain. Stick with the bodyweight basics here.

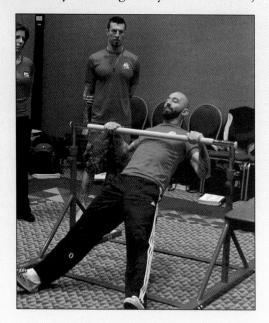

It's worth pointing out that most bodybuilders barely do any specialist work for the front and rear deltoid heads anyway. With all the heavy pulling and pushing these dudes do, these areas mass up without even needing any special attention—in fact, adding even more work in would probably be overkill. So instead, when most bodybuilders talk about training *shoulders*, they are really talking about work for the lateral head; that sacred side area that makes a dude's shoulders *wider*.

With this in mind, you can get a little creative. Static movements work the lateral deltoid well, and *safely* under load. Think of *handstands* and their variants: wall handstands, free handstands, asymmetrical handstands, one-arm handstands, etc. Walking on the hands is a fantastic deltoid movement which will swell up those cannonballs fast. I once worked out with a dude who claimed that the best shoulder exercise *in the world* was walking upstairs on your hands! If you can do that, you probably don't need any help from old Coach!

As I've gotten older, I've moved away from prison-style handstand presses against the wall and towards old school hand-balancing. Not only is hand balancing great for strength, size and coordination, it's also surprisingly easy on the shoulders, especially as you get a bit older. Plus, hand-balancing is a fun and interesting sport all by itself, aside from bodybuilding. If you want to learn more about this aspect of shoulder training, we are fortunate as hell to have the number one go-to guy in the whole world for hand-balancing as part of our PCC community: the calisthenics master Logan Christopher. Despite his tender age, Logan has been a very well-known and well respected expert in the strength and bodyweight community for many years. Go check out this guy's books, courses and DVDs on his site: *www.legendarystrength.com*. Logan not only has the best resources on hand-balancing and handstand pushups on this earth, but his back catalog of bodyweight and strength training material is just priceless. I'm not a "referrer" or any of that shit, and I get no money for saying this, but if you are serious about bodyweight you owe it to yourself to invest in some of that guy's teachings. You will not regret it.

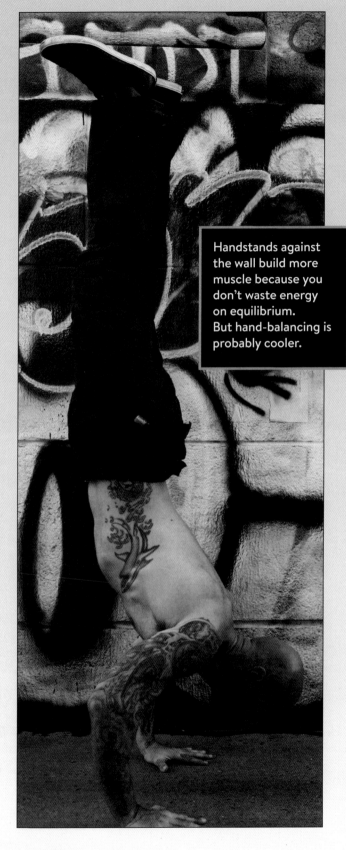

Handstands against the wall build more muscle because you don't waste energy on equilibrium. But hand-balancing is probably cooler.

AH'LL BE BACK

When training your back, the main thing to remember is that the back isn't a *bodypart*, so much as a *collection of bodyparts*. You got 4 major areas going on there:

1. The upper-back: *traps*
2. The mid-back: *rear deltoids, rhomboids* and *scapular (i.e., shoulder-blade) muscles*
3. The sides of the back: *lats*
4. The lower back/spinal muscles: *spinal erectors*

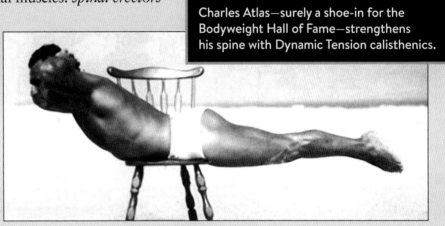

Charles Atlas—surely a shoe-in for the Bodyweight Hall of Fame—strengthens his spine with Dynamic Tension calisthenics.

Now, don't rush off and start working these different areas separately, willya my man? The body's muscles were designed to work as a *team*, and—provided you use the "big" compound exercises—you honestly don't need to work everything piecemeal. This is really where bodyweight shines—calisthenics makes your muscles pull in synergy better than any other method. For example, you might notice (a-hem) that the "Big Six" exercises I pimp in *Convict Conditioning* will work all these muscles (and more). The traps get a workout from *handstand pushups* and *bridging*; the mid-back and lats get worked by *horizontal pulls* and *pullups;* and nothing on earth works the spinal muscle like bridging does. But let's check out these areas a little closer.

LATS

Ah…pullups. Is there a finer "widener" in the bodybuilding world? Nope! I advise all athletes to make the vertical (upright) pullup the mainstay of their back training. This exercise will work the mid-back somewhat, but it works the lats like no other—even gym-addicted weight-trainers will head over to the pullup bar when they want to "get their lats back". This one's a no-brainer. All bodyweight bodybuilders should work with pullup progressions if they want to add maximum torso beef as fast and efficiently as possible.

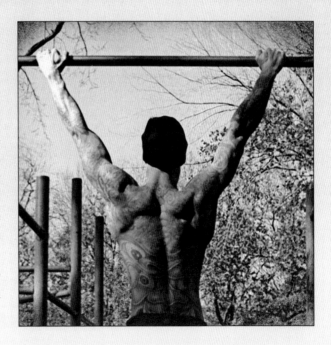

MID-BACK

Pullups alone will get you a long way. But as you become more advanced, you may wish to add in some kind of permanent *horizontal* pull to your upper-back routine. Why? Well, vertical pullups mainly work the *vertical* torso muscles—the lats. *Horizontal* pulling shifts more work onto the horizontal muscles of the back—the rear delts, scapular muscles and the lower heads of the trapezius. These are the "detail" muscles of the back, so loved by bodybuilders when they grow and thicken, resembling serpents swirling around the shoulder-blades.

I demand that all my students begin their personal training with a brutal regime of punishing, high-rep *horizontal* pulls. Why? Coz most men today—whether lifters or couch potatoes—are built back-to-front. They *reach forwards* constantly, whether bench pressing or net-surfing, or even just clicking the boob tube remote. They hardly ever *pull back*. As a result, their pushing muscles are switched on, while the antagonistic muscles of the upper back—which evolved to climb trees and should be strong as hell—are atrophied to nothing. No wonder so many modern folks have constant shoulder pain. The solution is an extended program of horizontal pull drills to set the system back to a healthy "default". Only then can the real progressive strength and mass-building begin, because only then is the shoulder girdle correctly balanced and primed.

Al Kavadlo calls horizontal pulls *Australian pullups* because you are "down under" the bar. (Last time I went down in a bar was in Yuba City in the 80s. She was a wild girl called Mariana… but I'll save that story for another time.) I place them *prior* to regular pullups in the *Convict Conditioning* progression for reasons I've already given, but Aussie pullups and vertical pullups can go hand-in-hand in the same routine.

Aussies can be trained progressively, like any other exercise. Begin with a high bar and your feet on the ground (imagine the opposite of *wall pushups*) and work your way up (or down?) to one-handed Aussie pullups, with your feet raised slightly higher than your hands. Real strength monsters can try Aussie pullups with *no* foot support—two-handed, from a front lever position. But you gotta be real powerful to try that shit. (Front and back levers are also incredible total-back exercises in their own right, but more on them in a little bit.)

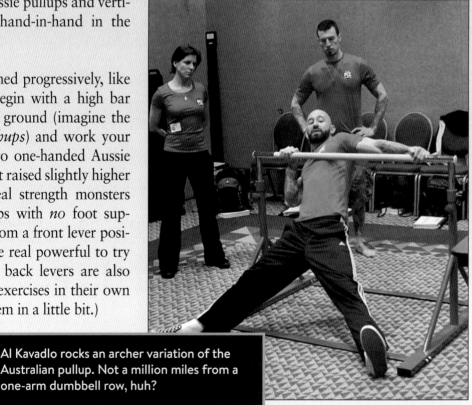

Al Kavadlo rocks an archer variation of the Australian pullup. Not a million miles from a one-arm dumbbell row, huh?

LOW BACK & SPINE

Many bodybuilders think only in terms of "low back" when working the spinal muscles, but this is a mistake: the *erector spinae* (spinal erectors) actually run all the way up the spine, from the hips to the skull. For this reason, just bending over with hip hinge-type motions cannot work the spinal muscles completely. You need to flex *all* the vertebrae to do this, and this can only be done with *bridging*. Not only does bridging fully work all the deep tissues of the spine, it also bullet-proofs the discs and—despite what some pencil-necks may tell you—it is also the safest spinal exercise because the discs are loaded while concave. As I said in *Convict Conditioning*:

> *"During bridges, the powerful spinal muscles are worked when the spine is arched back, which closes the joints. This is a very safe position, particularly if no external load is involved. Unfortunately, barbell exercises work the muscles with the spine rounded forwards, which opens the vertebrae, and puts the discs in danger of splitting or popping out. The leverage of the high external load as well as the convex opening of the vertebrae makes the back very vulnerable to injury during these barbell movements. The mighty Bruce Lee was performing barbell good mornings when he blew his back out badly in 1970. Doctors told him he would never perform kung fu again, but he trained himself back to full fitness—using calisthenics."*
>
> —Paul "Coach" Wade, Convict Conditioning, chapter 9

In *Convict Conditioning*, I teach the progressions leading to the ultimate form of the bridge for strength-mobility: the *stand-to-stand*. In stand-to-stands, you stand up straight, lean over backwards and place your palms on the floor, in a perfect bridge. From there, you lever yourself back up. Stand-to-stands are great, not least because they promote balance and coordination and you can use them as transitions to other exercises (bridge-to-handstand, handstand-to-bridge, etc). For building muscle, however, you might want to look at

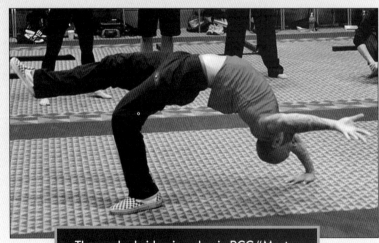

The gecko bridge is a classic PCC "Master Step", but Al makes it look easy as pie.

working towards *gecko bridges*—bridges where you support yourself using only one arm and the opposite leg. The static progressions to gecko bridges are taught in the PCC system, but you can also perform them dynamically, by pushing up and down from the floor. This is definitely best for muscle-building.

So bridging is a "must do". But there are other great exercises which work the spinal muscles. *Front levers* and *back levers* force the entire trunk to remain straight under the force of huge leverage, and this builds steely backs for sure. These are typically performed as static holds by bodyweight experts, but you can lever up into these positions for reps, bodybuilding-style. Back levers performed this way are particularly effective in building *huge* spinal strength and thickness.

In the **Convict Conditioning: Iron Spine** DVD I also gave instruction in a wonderful exercise, *inverse hyperextensions*. To perform these beauties, pop into a headstand, and—without bending your knees drastically—lower your toes to the floor. Then press your body straight again. This is a superb lower-back and spine exercise which requires zero equipment. (You can also do this technique from a handstand against a wall, but you need spinal muscles like the Terminator and total-body strength off the charts to do it. Very few bodybuilders could pull this off. So get practicing!)

One last tip…anybody who has been taught that deadlifting is the one-and-only posterior chain exercise needs to check out Al Kavadlo's now-classic article: *Bodyweight Deadlift Alternatives*. http://www.alkavadlo.com/2012/09/04/bodyweight-deadlift-alternatives/ (While you're there, check out the rest of his site. That guy is something awesome.)

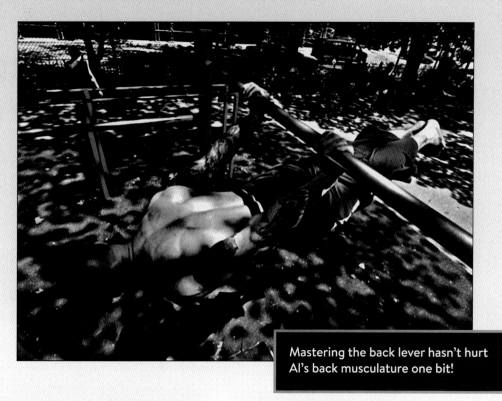

Mastering the back lever hasn't hurt Al's back musculature one bit!

CALVING SEASON

Calf-building theory, like forearms and neck, was thoroughly covered in *Convict Conditioning 2*. There's really nothing valuable to add to that, but I'll try and give you some basics in case you don't have the book. (You...you *will* go buy it though, right? Please. My electric bill is due, dude.)

Most writers of bodybuilding programs typically enjoin that calves should be trained by beginners, typically on leg day. I disagree. Guys working their legs on machines and with choppy barbell squats may not be training their calves, and probably need the extra work. But bodyweight athletes should be working towards the one-leg squat, and all calisthenics squatting progressions—being full and deep—work the entirety of the lower legs very well.

Full flat-footed squats—no blocks under those heels!—require optimal *tension-flexibility* (a.k.a. "supple strength") in the ankles and calves. The bent-ankle position at the bottom is called *dorsiflexion* by sports scientists, and it requires huge power in the shin muscles (*anterior tibialis*) to maintain, as well as all-round strength in the ankles and feet. Pushing up into a squat causes the ankles to straighten, strengthening the *soleus* and *gastrocnemius* muscles which make up the calf bulk. Deep, "ass-to-grass" squats on just *one leg* hugely magnify all these benefits to the calves, as well as adding functional balance and unilateral skill.

By the time you can perform twenty one-leg squats, your calves will be much more supple, more powerful, and your ankles/Achilles' tendon will be bulletproofed like friggin' steel cable. In addition, your calves will have grown in size, particularly if you were patient with progressions. For these reasons, whether you are an athlete, a strength trainer or a pure bodyweight bodybuilder, your first mission should be to gradually build to a full one-leg squat. Until you get there, you don't need to waste time on any specialist calf exercises. In fact, you might never need to specifically train your calves at all. Some men get true "diamond" calves just from one-leg squatting, and don't feel the need to add any further exercises.

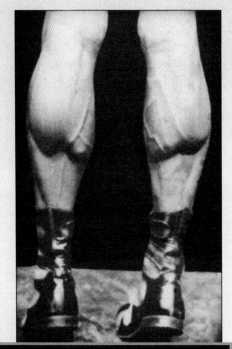

I just had to include this rare old school pic, also seen in CC2. Chanchal Prosad was an Indian muscle-control expert in the 30's. These calves were built using bodyweight only!

Just as with forearm growth, genetics plays a role in calf development; not just growth potential, but also factors like muscle length. For example some brothers have "shorter" calves; meaning the belly of the large calf muscle, the gastrocnemius, is short and stubby. This is often true of athletes of African heritage. If you look at a black bodybuilder like Tony Pearson, you'll notice that although all his muscles are hugely developed, his calves are like tennis balls stuck just below his knee. No matter how big he builds them, there's just not enough muscle there to expand very much. This is a generalization, naturally; some black bodybuilders have long, full calves; Sergio Oliva comes to mind. Nor are short calves a problem when it comes to athleticism. Many fine sprinters have short calves—what makes the ankles powerful is not the calf size, but the elasticity of the long Achilles' tendon. I've heard some people argue that short calves are actually *better* for athleticism! But not for bodybuilding, right?

If you do want to add specific calf exercises to your program, bodyweight calf raises are a good choice. Many people consider bodyweight too light to stress the calves into growth, but these folks are forgetting that the calves carry the body around all day—they have evolved to handle a tremendous volume of work, and for this reason they need high reps (sometimes in the hundreds) to really grow. So you should look at bodyweight calf raises as an opportunity to *strictly* explore these higher rep ranges.

That doesn't mean you can't be progressive. You can begin with calf raises off the floor, and move to fuller raises with your heels hanging off a step; you can move from two legs to one leg; from straight knees to bent knees, etc. All these variables will add difficulty. I show you how to construct a linear series of progressions using these "tougheners" in *Convict Conditioning 2*.

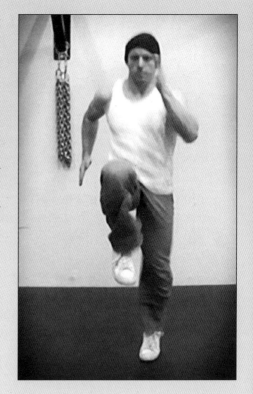

The calves are naturally explosive muscles, and explosive bodyweight work is very good for calf-building. I'm talking:

* Sprints
* Box jumps
* Hill sprints (especially)
* Dead leaps
* Plyometric jumps
* Tuck jumps

...and so on. A really good tip is to mix-n-match slow *and* explosive work for calves. Here's a good example of such a "shock" workout: when I was on the inside, I occasionally performed strict, deep, slow double-leg calf raises off a stack of books, aiming for a hundred reps. When I got to a twenty my calves were burning, when I got to fifty they were in agony, and by a hundred I was close to screaming! Despite the ache and pain, when I reached triple figures I would immediately step off the books and—knees together—hop up and down as high as possible for about sixty seconds (if I could make it). A minute seemed like forever, and by the time it was up, you better believe that my calves had taken in a better workout than lifting a thousand pounds on a heavy-duty gym machine! I could barely hop an inch. But I still wasn't finished. I would immediately start jogging on the spot, fast as possible, aiming at sixty seconds again. I never made it—I usually just collapsed on the floor at about thirty seconds, clutching my swollen calves. All bodybuilders who think squatting heavy weights is the only measure of a man should take a shot at this nightmare!

You should only try this type of crazy shit if you are conditioned to it, but it works. Methods like this are so brutal (and effective) that they can put an inch or more on stubborn calves in just weeks. If you can train like this just once a week for a few months, you better get ready to outgrow your socks, boy.

TNT: TOTAL NECK AND TRAPS

Hold it. Do bodybuilders even need to do neck work? Mebbe yes, mebbe no. A well-developed neck—like forearms and calves—is often one of those genetic gifts delivered by the Big Man upstairs. If you have a pencil where that neck is though, you might want to get cracking. At the very least, chicks dig a strong-looking, muscular neck...as long as you don't go too far and start looking like Bluto. (What the fu...you don't know who *Bluto* is?! Millenials. Get the f*** out of my sight.)

I've always thought it was kinda weird that the neck is the most exposed bodypart on a day-to-day basis, yet bodybuilders are less likely to train the neck than any other set of muscles. Classically-minded bodybuilders, concerned with aesthetics, need a well-developed neck, kept in perfect proportion to the rest of the body. Leonardo da Vinci, master of symmetry, determined (from his reading of classical sources) that on the perfect human body, the neck should be the same girth as the *upper arms* and *calves*. There is no pro bodybuilder in the world today with that kinda perfection of proportion. Some of the old-timers were able to achieve it, however, most notably 1947 Mr America, Steve Reeves, who proudly boasted and 18 inch neck to go with his 18 inch arms and calves.

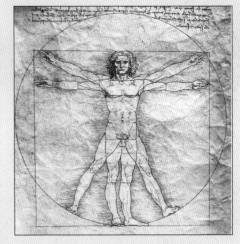

Reeves was arguably one of the most perfectly-built men in history, and his look was so balanced, so *right*, he broke into the movies—becoming the highest paid actor in Europe, for a while. Remember, this was in the 1950s—years before the world was accustomed to the look of bodybuilders on the big screen. Yet Reeves was admired by men and adored by women because his build was perfectly proportioned. His neck had something to do with that.

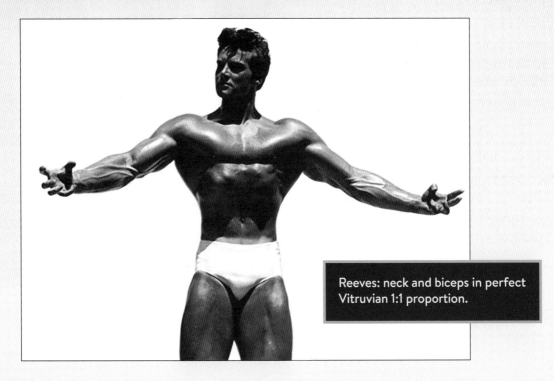

Reeves: neck and biceps in perfect Vitruvian 1:1 proportion.

Beginners should get adequate neck and trapezius work from exercises like bridges and inversions such as headstands and handstands. Handstands certainly are an elite-level technique for developing the upper trapezius muscles between the neck and shoulders; some of the most impressive traps on the planet belong to male gymnasts, because they spend half their lives upside-down on their hands. Walking on the hands is another wonderful exercise for the traps, developing them from all angles.

Most gym-going bodybuilders rely on straining with barbell and dumbbell shrugs to specialize on their traps, but an equally effective variant exists for their bodyweight brothers: *handstand shrugs*. Get into a handstand against the wall, and perform a good, deep shrug of the shoulders. The movement will be difficult, short and choppy at first, but over time you will gain a full range-of-motion. By the time you can perform two sets of twenty deep, slow reps, your traps will look like frigging cans of beans.

If you want more *neck*, and filling out your collar is something you want to explore, forget those decapitation machines in the gym, or those headache-inducing head straps. Those things are all total crap. The safest, most natural and most productive techniques for building a bull-nape are the most primal ones, used religiously by grapplers and boxers since time immemorial. I'm talking a hardcore diet of *wrestler's bridges*—front, back, and side. If you want a fully detailed masterclass in totally dominating these ancient techniques, it's all in **Convict Conditioning 2**. I should know, I left it there for ya.

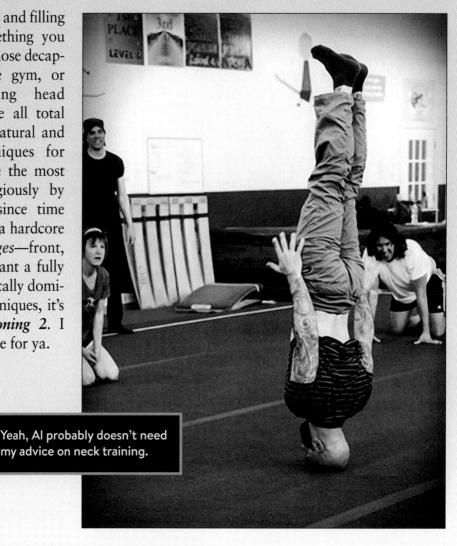

Yeah, Al probably doesn't need my advice on neck training.

4

Okay.
Now Gimme a
Program

Whenever I start talking to folks about applying calisthenics to bodybuilding, I inevitably wind up getting asked the following practical question: *what kind of routine should* I use?

The answer should be obvious—a *bodybuilding* routine!

If you want to pack on muscle using bodyweight, it's no good training like a *gymnast* or a *martial artist* or a *dancer* or a *yoga expert*, no matter how impressive those *skill-based* practitioners might be at performing advanced calisthenics. You need a different mindset. You need to train like a *bodybuilder*! The only difference between you and the bodybuilders in the gym is that they use tools like barbells and dumbbells; for you, your body must become your tool-kit. Your body must become your gym, stud!

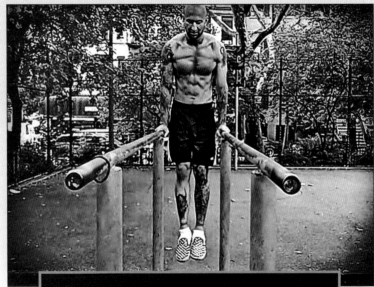

Al Kavadlo can use parallel bars, horizontal bars, or just the floor when he works out.

This book is meant to be a primer on bodyweight bodybuilding *theory*, so listing dozens of programs isn't gonna be too helpful. It'll be more useful to discuss some basic *principles* behind programming, with a few examples, so you can do your own programming. *Teach a guy to fish*, and all that bullshit, eh?

THE PROGRAMMING LINE: SIMPLE TO COMPLEX

The most important thing to understand about bodybuilding routines is that they tend to follow a simple linear procession. At one end you have programs with *minimum* complexity, and at the other end you have programs with *maximum* complexity. We might call this *the programming line*, and picture it on a basic graph like this:

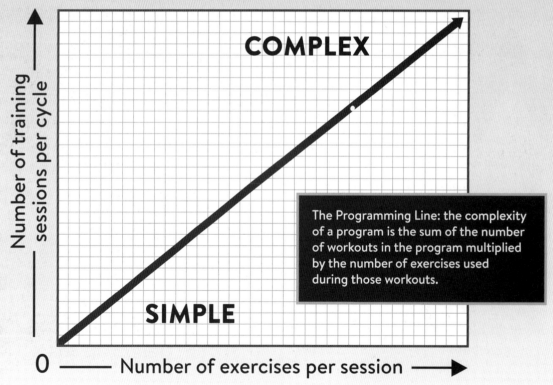

PROGRAMMING LINE STATUS:

COMPLEX

SIMPLE

Number of training sessions per cycle

0 —— Number of exercises per session ——>

The Programming Line: the complexity of a program is the sum of the number of workouts in the program multiplied by the number of exercises used during those workouts.

Every training program falls somewhere in this graph, with most "classic" bodybuilding routines lying somewhere on the line.

Simple programs with **minimum** complexity feature:

- Fewer training sessions per cycle
- Fewer exercises per training session
- Typically more compound (or multi-joint) exercises:

By contrast, programs with **maximum** complexity feature:

- More training sessions per cycle
- More exercises per training session
- Typically more isolation (or single-joint) exercises

As a rule, beginners are advised to follow the simpler programs, while intermediate and advanced bodybuilders will use more complex programs.

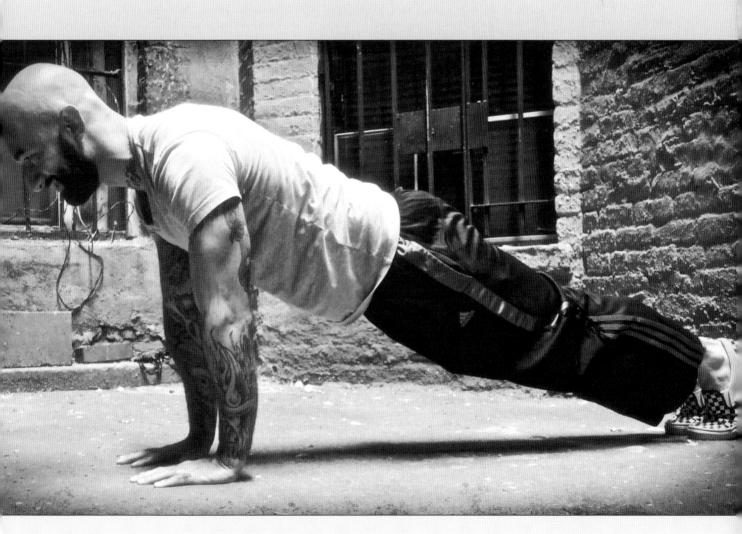

SIMPLE BEATS COMPLEX!

So what should you choose? A simple program with a few basic exercises and limited workouts, or a complex program with lots of workouts and a longer roll call of techniques? Which is better?

There's no question that beginner athletes always want to rush ahead and use more complex programs. They check out the complex routines featured in magazines, and try to follow them. They seem glamorous, interesting—and besides, if they follow an advanced routine they'll be more advanced, right?

In reality—not muscle magazines or the gym, but ACTUAL physiological reality—they should be following the opposite course. As a general rule, *you should always follow simpler programs if you can*. Why? Three VERY important reasons:

REASON 1: ADDED FREQUENCY

Fewer training sessions per cycle means that *the same exercises are worked more often*. This gives more opportunity for progress. Think about a guy working the VERY simple program on page 62—just squats, pushups and pullups three or four times per week. There is just ONE session per cycle—one workout every two/three days. He is working his pullups (for example) three or four times a week. Compare that to an advanced guy on the complex 3-way split routine given on page 67. He might be doing more total work, but he is only doing his pullups once every fivedays. Who is going to progress faster?

REASON 2: SUPERIOR FOCUS

Fewer exercises per training session means that focus and energy aren't spread over lots and lots of techniques, but is poured exclusively into just a few exercises. This makes progress incredibly rapid. Ask yourself: who is going to put more energy into their pullups? The guy who is doing pullups, or the guy who is doing pullups plus another five exercises? It's simple thermodynamics—your body only has so much energy to go around. The more you condense that energy into a few useful exercises, the better you will get at those valuable exercises—and that's the name of the game, kid.

REASON 3: INCREASED EFFICIENCY

Simple routines tend to be built around bigger, compound, multi-joint exercises; while complex routines also include single-joint exercises intended for isolation of individual muscles. Almost by definition, multi-joint exercises build more muscle, because they work multiple muscles in unison; they also teach the body to work in a more coordinated manner, increasing strength faster and in turn allowing more stress to be thrown on the muscles during future training. In layman's terms, working more with compound exercises gives an athlete a bigger bang for his buck—every time.

That's it. Simple programs—basic workouts, fewer exercises, and a priority for the big compound exercises—is always what you should be shooting for. Hands down.

WHEN TO MOVE UP THE PROGRAMMING LINE..?

If simpler, more basic routines are always the best, why do advanced bodybuilders tend to follow more complex routines? Programs with different sessions for different bodyparts, with dozens of exercises, and so on? Several points to mull over:

• OLD SCHOOL

Advanced bodybuilders don't all follow super-complex routines. Many stick to the most basic routines, and thrive on them. This was certainly true in the old days (when men were more accustomed to work!) and top bodybuilders like John Grimek, Steve Reeves and Reg Park used simple routines where they trained the whole body with basics, three times per week.

• PRE-CONTEST CONFUSION

Even successful modern bodybuilders probably train with simpler programs than you think. The mega-extended split routines you see in the magazines or on the net are usually *pre-contest* routines designed to put the finishing touches on a physique—they're not meant to put on real mass. So why print them? They make the athletes look more sophisticated! In truth, even bodybuilders who do use complex programs often return to the simpler routines from time to time, when they need to grow faster.

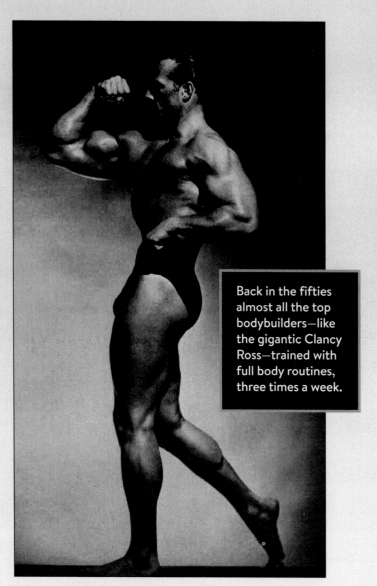

Back in the fifties almost all the top bodybuilders—like the gigantic Clancy Ross—trained with full body routines, three times a week.

• REDUCED FREQUENCY

Believe it or not, the bigger and more advanced a bodybuilder becomes, the less they are able to train. A beginner bodybuilder bench pressing a hundred pounds can possibly get away with benching three times per week. A man who benches 500 pounds? No way! It's too much strain on the joints, soft tissues and recovery system. As mentioned earlier, more complex programs actually feature LESS frequent training—especially on the big compound exercises—allowing for more recovery when performed correctly.

• DIMINISHING RETURNS

Advanced men also suffer the natural phenomena of *diminishing returns*—the more they develop their bodies, the harder it is to gain any more muscle over time. So they shift from the trusted basic, simple routines—which are giving them less results—and explore other variables, like more volume, more exercises, different exercises, etc. in the hope that the added complexity will stimulate more growth. (Whether this actually works or is purely psychological is another matter!)

• "ANGULAR" TRAINING

Typically, highly advanced bodybuilders who have trained for 10+ years have built a level of mass close to their body's limit. When this happens, they often ease back on the basics, and add more exercises to hit their muscles from every possible angle, hoping to actualize their full potential, fill in any weak points, and eke out that last bit of "shape" that eluded them when training solely with basic moves.

• VARIETY

Boredom and stress are also reasons athletes begin using more complex programs. Hard, progressive work on the basics is tough! Adding in exercises and spreading effort over more volume can actually be a lot easier, and certainly more interesting from time-to-time than the brutal basics.

The take-home message is—always use the simplest program you can get away with—it will make you bigger and stronger faster than more complex shit. However, there are *some* valid reasons to move up the programming line and explore more complex programs. Unless you already have all the muscle mass you want—and need to start performing the finishing touches on an already massive physique—the best reason is to *avoid overtraining*. When you gain strength and the simplest routines, like the total-body workout on page 63, are too much for you to handle, move to an upper-body/lower body routine (page 64). This can last an athlete years and years.

PROGRAM TEMPLATES, BITCHES!

There are more sophisticated approaches to programming in *Convict Conditioning*, but I'll outline a few fundamental templates here. Why? Because I like ya. I think you're cool, and I like your hair. Also, I want you to grow, kid.

- A note for new fish: you should be aware that the exercises given are meant to be bodyweight *progressions*. So where it says *pushup progression*, for example, it means that you should be doing *increasingly tougher* types of pushup as you get stronger. Where do you learn these progressions? A great start would be to go to the PCC blog: *pccblog.dragondoor.com*. Engage with the community there, and check out the archive or articles lovingly compiled by the wonderful girya girl, Adrienne Harvey PCC. Good books to learn progressions would include *Convict Conditioning 1 & 2* or Al Kavadlo's great *Pushing the Limits!* Or *Raising the Bar.*

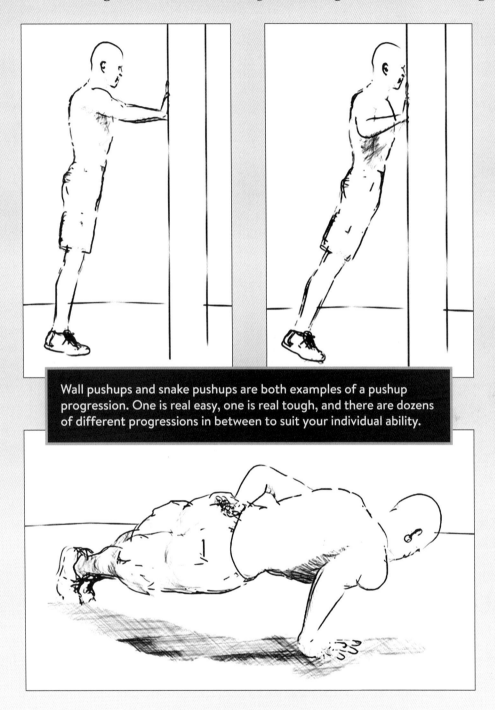

Wall pushups and snake pushups are both examples of a pushup progression. One is real easy, one is real tough, and there are dozens of different progressions in between to suit your individual ability.

- You might also notice that some of these templates don't list exercise techniques—instead they might just list a bodypart, like *triceps exercise*. That means you get to choose what exercises to perform for that area. Don't panic if you're not sure. If you are hankering after some numero uno quality bodyweight exercises I've included a bunch for each bodypart in chapter 3: *"Coach" Wade's Bodypart Tactics.* Cool, daddio.

TOTAL BODY 1

Day 1:   Squat progression
                Pullup progression
                Pushup progression

Day 2:   Off

Repeat

NB: Unless you are a total novice using very easy progressions, even this might be too much work. Many athletes would be better off just repeating DAY 1 on Mondays, Wednesdays and Fridays, with Weekends completely off for recovery.

PROGRAMMING LINE STATUS:

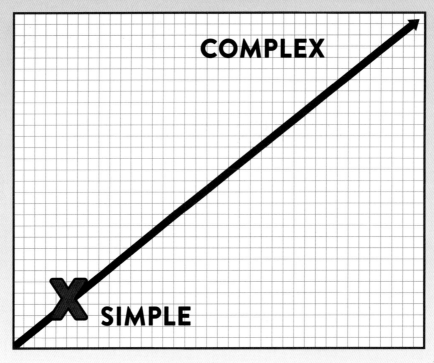

TOTAL BODY 2

Day 1:   Squat progression
                Pushup progression
                Sit-up progression
                Pullup progression
                Bridge progression
                Inversion progression (e.g., handstand)

Day 2:   Off

Repeat

PROGRAMMING LINE STATUS:

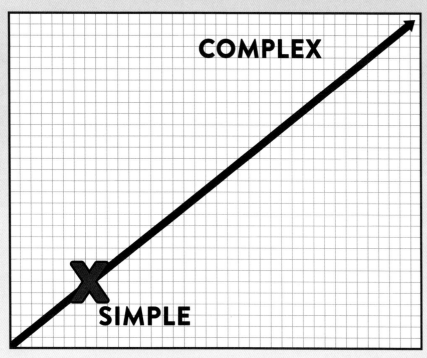

UPPER/LOWER-BODY SPLIT 1

Day 1:   Pushup progression
          Pullup progression
          Inversion progression (e.g., handstand pushup)

Day 2:   Squat progression
          Bridge progression
          Leg raise progression

Day 3:   Off

Repeat

PROGRAMMING LINE STATUS:

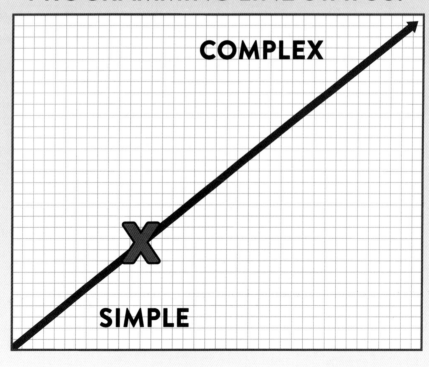

UPPER/LOWER-BODY SPLIT 2

Day 1:   Pushup progression
               Pullup progression
               Handstand pushup progression
               Australian pullup progression

Day 2:   Off

Day 3:   Calf exercise
               Squat progression
               Bridge progression
               Leg raise progression

Day 4:   Off

Repeat

PROGRAMMING LINE STATUS:

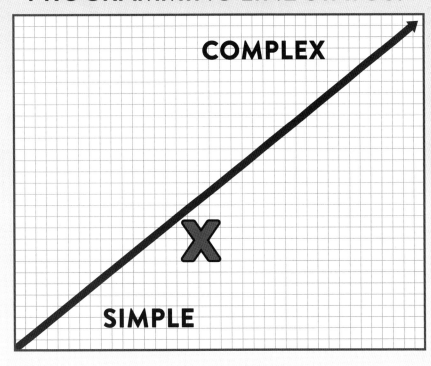

COMPLEX

X

SIMPLE

3-WAY SPLIT 1

Day 1:   Handstand Pushup
          progression
          Pushup progression
          Biceps exercise
          Hang grip progression

Day 2:   Squat progression
          Bridge progression
          Leg raise progression
          Calf exercise

Day 3:   Pullup progression
          Australian pullup
          progression
          Triceps exercise
          Fingertip pushup
          progression

Day 4:   Off

Repeat

PROGRAMMING LINE STATUS:

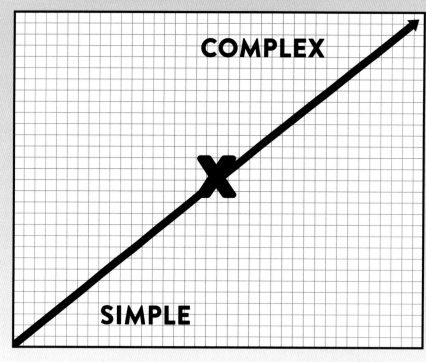

COMPLEX

SIMPLE

3-WAY SPLIT 2

Day 1:   Pushup progression
          Handstand pushup progression
          Dips
          Triceps exercise
          Fingertip progression

Day 2:   Off

Day 3:   Pullup progression
          Australian pullup progression
          Muscle-Up work
          Biceps exercise
          Hang grip progression

Day 4:   Squat progression
          Bridge progression
          Leg raise progression
          Box jumps or sprints
          Calf work

Day 5:   Off

Repeat

PROGRAMMING LINE STATUS:

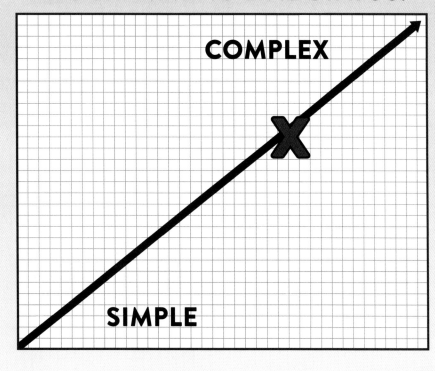

COMPLEX

X

SIMPLE

4-WAY SPLIT 1

Day 1:   Pushup exercise 1
         Handstand pushup
            progression
         Pushup exercise 2
         Shoulder exercise 2
         Neck work

Day 2:   Midsection work
         Calf work
         Squat progression
         Quad exercise
         Hamstring exercise
         Sprints/jumps

Day 3:   Pullup Progression
         Horizontal pullup
            progression
         Bridges
         Another bar exercise

Day 4:   Biceps Work
         Triceps work
         Grip/forearm work

Day 5:   Off

Repeat

PROGRAMMING LINE STATUS:

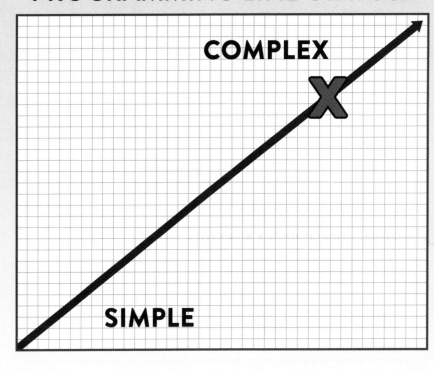

4-WAY SPLIT 2

Day 1:   Calf work
          Hamstring exercise
          Squat progression
          Quad exercise
          Midsection work
          Sprints/jumps

Day 2:   Pushup exercise 1
          Pushup exercise 2
          Dips
          Triceps exercise
          Fingertip training
          Deep breathing exercises

Day 3:   Lever training
          Pullup Exercise 1
          Pullups exercise 2
          Horizontal pullup progression
          Biceps exercise
          Bridges

Day 4:   Hand-balancing
          Shoulder exercise 2
          Neck work
          Grip exercise 1
          Grip exercise 2

Day 5: Off

Repeat

PROGRAMMING LINE STATUS:

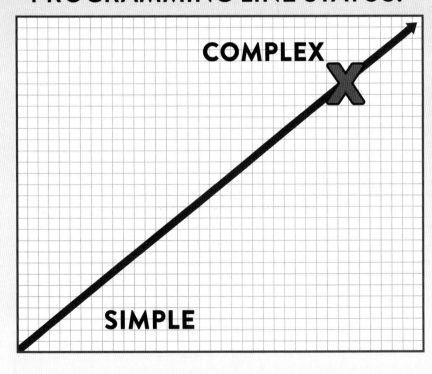

COMPLEX

SIMPLE

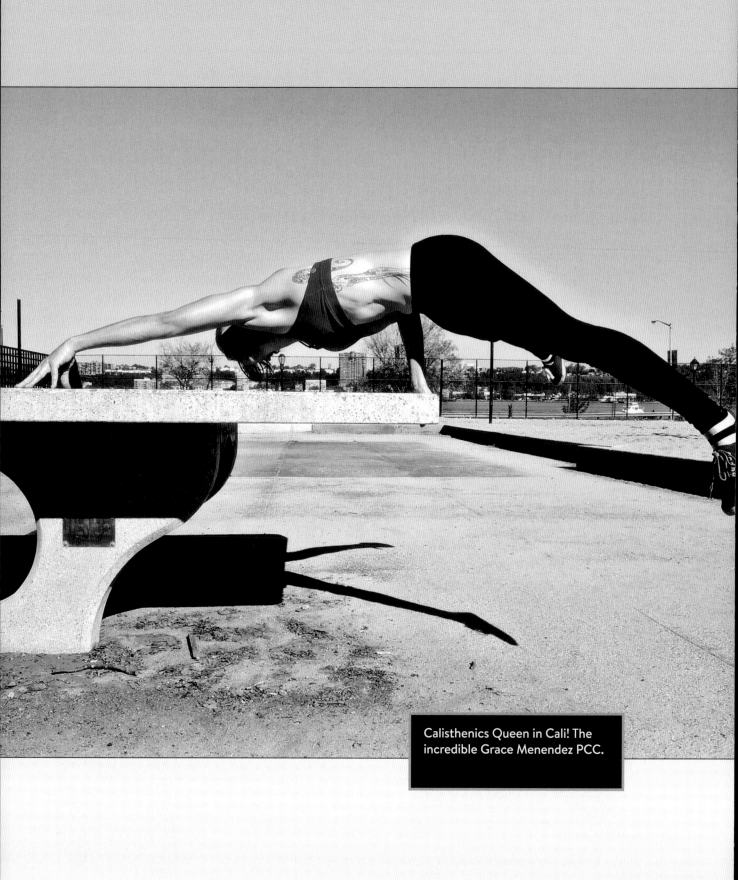

Calisthenics Queen in Cali! The incredible Grace Menendez PCC.

C-MASS — CALISTHENICS MASS

5

TROUBLESHOOTING MUSCLE-GROWTH: THE FAQ

Well there you go…70 pages of stone cold truth on how to pack your frame with slabs of dense muscle, using old school calisthenics.

But you can't handle the truth!

…huh? Whazzat? You *can* handle the truth, but you got a couple questions? Okay dude, my bad. Fire away.

Q. Why bodyweight? Why can't I use weights and machines to build muscle?

A. You can. You can easily apply the concepts and principles outlined in this manual to work with weights and resistance machines. You can use them to build muscle using sandbags or stacks of bricks if you like. The PCC organization is simply focused on bodyweight work. Speaking personally, I believe that training with bodyweight *blows external weights away* in terms of overall training benefits, for the reasons I gave in my book, **Convict Conditioning**.

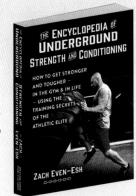

If you really wanna explore external weights, the best book on functional, old-school athletic strength and power is *The Encyclopedia of Underground Strength and Conditioning*, by the awesome Zach Even-Esh. Check it out!

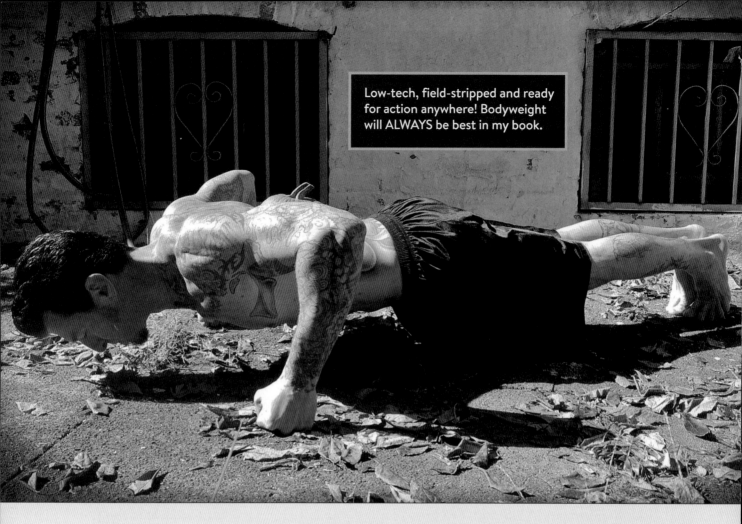

Low-tech, field-stripped and ready for action anywhere! Bodyweight will ALWAYS be best in my book.

Q. I understand that pull-ups and chin-ups are superior exercises for building muscle in the lats and biceps. Unfortunately I cannot yet perform pull-ups. Should I use assistance bands instead?

A. Athletes have been working towards pullups for thousands of years before assistance bands were invented. You do not need them. Until you are strong enough for regular pullups, why not work with *Australian pullups*? Check out this unbeatable video from our dynamite Lead Instructor, Al Kavadlo: *http://www.alkavadlo.com/2010/01/07/all-about-australian-pull-ups/*

You can make Australian pullups harder and harder over time, as Al shows in the vid.

Australian pullups are a horizontal movement, but you can also gain strength progressively with vertical pulling movements. The PCC Instructor's Manual includes nearly seventy vertical pull-up variations! If you are nearly ready for true pullups, howabout *jackknife pull-ups*? With jackknife pullups you rest your heels on a box or base to assist you with the upwards motion.

With moves like these, you don't need bands.

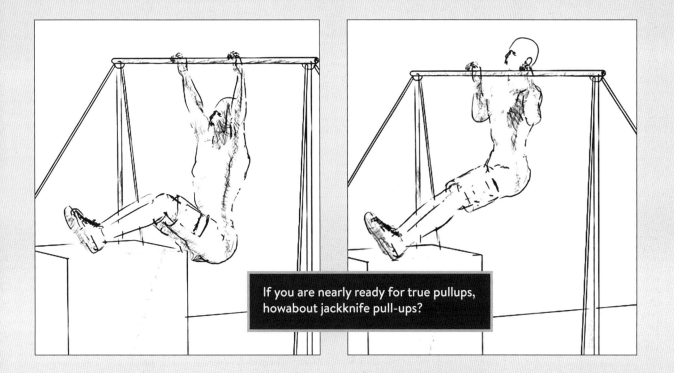

If you are nearly ready for true pullups, howabout jackknife pull-ups?

Q. Looking at gymnasts, I have no doubt that progressive calisthenics methods can build a huge upper body. But what about the legs? Won't it leave me with stick legs?

A. Nah, there are plenty of bodyweight leg training techniques, as I mentioned in chapter three. It's sad but true, but most of the guys who diss on bodyweight leg work are either fat and useless or skinny theorizers who never took a bodyweight workout in their lives.

Once you can do two sets of twenty strict one-leg squats, the same in gecko bridges, followed by a 25 inch vertical jump, then come back and tell me calisthenics is no good for your wheels. Otherwise, what the hell are you waiting for?

Q. Coach, can you name the exercises that belong into an abbreviated routine for a total beginner? Which are the most essential without leaving gaps in my ability?

A. For a rank beginner? A pullup, a pushup, a squat, a leg raise. As you gain strength, add inverse positions and bridges. When you feel comfortable again, you can add more; perhaps a horizontal pulling movement, such as Australian pullups or front levers.

Q. *"Big" bodyweight exercises such as push-ups and pull-ups may target the larger muscles of the body (pecs, lats, biceps, etc.), but what about the smaller muscles which are still so important to the bodybuilder? Things like forearms, the calves, the neck?*

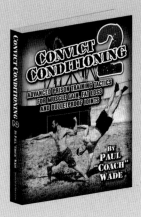

A. I covered this question fully in my book, *Convict Conditioning 2*. The forearms are to be worked with progressive bodyweight hangs and progressive fingertip pushups, amongst other exercises. The calves can be worked with standing or squatting calf raises, both of which can be made progressive—and finished off with explosive jumping-style movements. Progressive wrestler's bridges and frontal neck bridges will build a neck bigger and more functional than anything built with weights.

I've said it before and I'll say it again—there is *no* muscle, or set of muscles, which you can work with weights or machines that cannot be worked—more efficiently!—with your own bodyweight. You just need to know *how*.

Q. *I have been told I need to use a weighted vest on my push-ups and pull-ups if I want to get stronger and gain muscle. Is this true?*

A. No—you don't need a vest. In fact, far from helping athletes, weighted vests hold them back. Instead of moving from an exercise they can perform, to a tougher step, vest-users just sling on the vest and stay with the same exercise, never blossoming or increasing their skill-base by exploring newer, more difficult techniques. Vests also screw up your form—maybe only slightly, but they do.

That said—many other trainers will disagree. If your heart says play with the vest do it—you might have some fun. But do you NEED it? *Nah!*

Q. *Is bodyweight training suitable for women? Do you know of any women who achieved the "Master Steps" laid out in Convict Conditioning?*

Women cannot gain size like the dudes can due to much lower testosterone levels. Doesn't mean they can't get strong as all shit though! There's no doubt about it—females respond just as well to strength calisthenics as men. There are several reasons for this. Some of it has to do with the fact that calisthenics is about proportional strength, and women are generally lighter than their ball-laden counterparts. Some of it has to do with the natural joint mobility females enjoy (and which increases during pregnancy). A lot of it is due to simple aesthetics; typically, women are more drawn to body movement (think dance, gymnastics) than to big, ugly, rusty weights.

As for the Master Steps, there are numerous female contenders. I often talk about the achievements of old-time male athletes, but I'm guilty of neglecting the women of the field, who were just as amazing—or more. Lillian Leitzel (born 1890s) was an acrobat at Barnum's circus who could bust out nearly thirty one-arm pullups. The 19th Century Welsh strongwoman Vulcana could allegedly perform a one-arm handstand pushup. (At age 13 she also wrestled down and captured a runaway stallion!) So yes—a woman CAN get there.

YOU can get there!

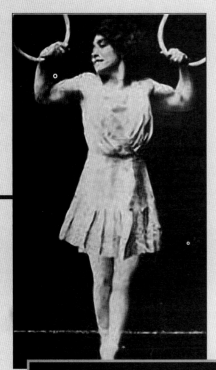

The Legendary Lillian Leitzel. Check out the guns!

Q. I am very interested in gaining size—not just muscle mass, but also height. Is it possible that calisthenics can increase my height?

It's not just possible—I've seen it done on multiple occasions. In the old days, there was an entire sub-discipline of calisthenics devoted to increasing height. It was seen as important as muscle growth—and why the hell not? In fact, experience has shown that height can be maintained and even increased by a couple of inches (or more) over time. The keys are:

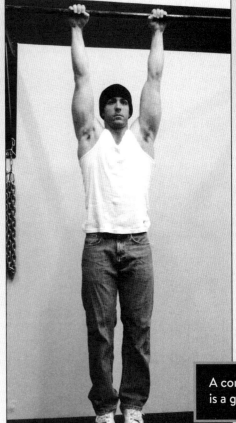

A compressed spine is shorter than a relaxed one. Simple hanging is a great way to relax your spine after a tough workout.

- Don't compress your spine. Avoid regular heavy squats, deadlifts, leg presses, etc. If you run or jump, don't overdo it.

- Use good posture daily. Keep your spine elongated (imagine your head is pulled up by a cable) and your chest subtly up and out.

- Train the discs: keep them healthy and regenerating—bridging every week!

- Decompress the spine after bridging with forward bends.

- Maximum height requires strong bones, and strong bones require calcium. You don't need to go overboard with supplements, but don't avoid dairy if you want to optimize your height.

Specialist exercises include:

1. **Standing postures:** emphasizing height and upwards stretch
2. **Back bends** for health/growth of the spine/discs
3. **Forward bends** to stretch out/decompress the discs
4. **Spinal twists** to loosen over-tight spines and rib structures
5. **Deep breathing** to expand the ribcage

Does this approach work? Most guys lose an inch or so as they get older. In my mid-fifties I'm the same height I was when I was 21. I'm convinced bridging is the reason. I doubt there are any heavy weight-lifters or bodybuilders who can say the same. Look at Arnold—he's shrunk like a motherf***er over the years.

For more information on this topic, I totally recommend the old manual *Yoga for the Athlete* by Harvey Day—if you can find a copy. There is an excellent chapter on calisthenics for height.

Q. You have said that moving exercises are superior to isometrics when it comes to mass gain. I am interested in getting huge shoulders, but Convict Conditioning gives several static (isometric) exercises early on in the handstand pushup chain. Can you give me any moving exercises I can use instead, to work up to handstand pushups?

A. Sure. Just remember that inverse (upside-down) work is stressful on the soft tissues of the shoulders and elbows. Before you even consider hard inverse work, make sure you have put your time in with regular, flat pushups, to toughen up these areas. After that:

- Decline pushups
- Pike pushups
- Low base (knee height) jackknife pushups
- Jackknife (hip/upper thigh height) pushups

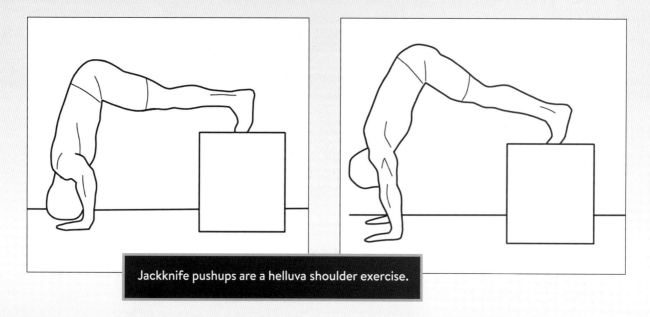

Jackknife pushups are a helluva shoulder exercise.

From there you can move straight to handstand pushups against a wall. Another alternative is old-fashioned "Marion pushups". They involve wedging your feet against a wall while busting out pushups with hands flat on the floor. Give yourself a goal (say, 10-15 reps) and each time you reach the goal—perfect form, Jack—you raise the feet by an inch or so. Keep track of your progress with chalk or a pen line. Cheap, simple, and real powerful if you get it right.

Q. I have heard that the teenage years are the ideal age for building muscle. Is there any point in trying to build muscle after the age of forty?

A. This is nonsense—pure bullshit. The current thinking on age and strength-performance has been completely skewed by the presence of performance-enhancing drugs. Modern professional bodybuilders (and many other pro sportsmen and women) begin taking drugs in their teens, and by the age of forty or fifty, their bodies are completely burnt out. In the real (drug-free) world, teenagers typically possess metabolisms so fast that building muscle is incredibly difficult. By the late thirties/early forties, the metabolism has slowed down radically, while testosterone levels are still at their highest. As a result these are the golden years for building muscle!

True, kick-ass strength in the fifties and sixties is not a problem. Many of the old-time strongmen could perform their awe-inspiring acts in their EIGHTIES. Drug-free athletes of the modern era should forget the bullshit fed to them by the modern, steroid-fuelled sporting world, and readjust their attitudes to the old school, SUPERIOR standards.

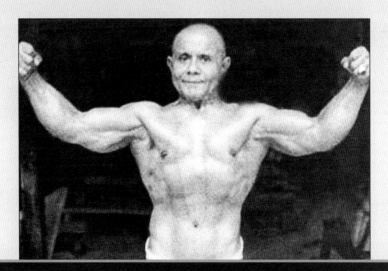

Manohar Aich was born in Bangladesh in 1913. After nearly dying of black fever, Manohar rebuilt himself using calisthenics; pushups, pullups, bodyweight squats and leg raises. By his own estimate, he built most of his physique with bodyweight work, and only began weight-training in his thirties. He has never touched bodybuilding drugs. He is 75 in the above photo. At the time of writing, Manohar is over a hundred years old, and he still exercises daily. He competed in his last bodybuilding competition at the age of 90. He is living proof that if you protect your joints with calisthenics, and build your hormonal profile without resorting to steroids, you can build muscle throughout your lifetime.

Q. I have had some knee problems in the past; any tips for keeping my knee joints healthy so I can build more leg mass?

A. Very, very common question. Knee care should be an issue all athletes look at—no matter how young they are. Here are six pointers to keep in mind for mega-knee health:

1. Avoid ponderous poundages. Huge squats and deadlifts may be all the rage now, but I've spoken to literally hundreds of older heavy squatters, and their knees are ALL f***ed up. To a man. Stick to bodyweight.

2. Depth is key for all tendon strengthening. You need to support your weight with knees *fully* bent. Building to deep one-leg squats will give you knees of iron—but get there slowly!

3. The hamstrings and calves also support the knee joint—not just the quads. Everyone should be bridging for knee health, and dudes with unstable knees should learn to love one-leg calf work!

4. The knee gets its nutrition largely from synovial fluid. This tends to be circulated when you "open" the joint by circling it. Lift your foot off the floor and circle the knee (never circle your knees with feet on the floor, as you see martial artists do. The knee is a hinge joint, and isn't meant to be circled under weight).

5. These days folks eat meat off the bone, but avoid "gristle"—which is cartilage. As a result, modern humans all have bad joints. To help out, they are taking shit like glucosamine, which is...ta daa! Basically cartilage. Eat your gristle now and again if you want to build strong cartilage!

6. I HATE recommending supplements, but you know what? Fish oil really seems to help the knees. It actually works.

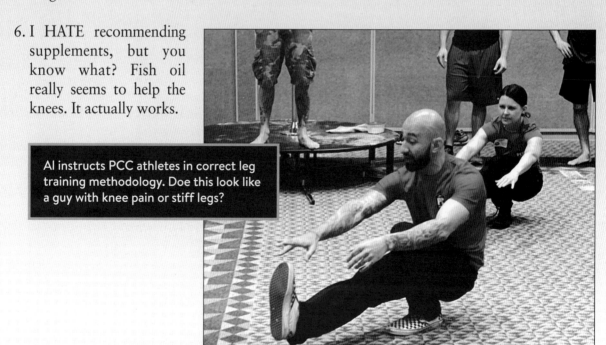

Al instructs PCC athletes in correct leg training methodology. Doe this look like a guy with knee pain or stiff legs?

Q. I'm pretty skinny and I have always had a huge amount of trouble putting on weight—any weight, even fat. Building muscle is virtually impossible for me. What program should I be on?

A. Believe it or not, the program you follow isn't as important as the PRINCIPLES and the LIFESTYLE you adopt. Here's what you do:

1. Keep a log. Use a solid program like *Hard Time*. Begin a step or so down from your usual exercises, and seek to make progress every week—by at least one rep. Really push yourself.

1.b. At the end of your upper body workout, explore dips (warm up then two hard sets). If you don't have a parallel bar, look to straight bar dips. These are a real torso/triceps builder.

2. Make this a short-term project—to keep you motivated. I want an inch on those arms in four months!

3. Eat four times a day. LIKE CLOCKWORK. Three meals, one snack. Eat a big meal when you sit down, featuring plenty of carbs, fats and protein. Favor ground beef, hamburger, sausage, eggs, etc. Really load up. Don't be afraid of junk. (If you drink on weekends that's cool, but stick to beer over spirits. More carbs—it'll slow down your metabolism too. Many old-time strongmen used to train on beer. I said "if" you drink, Jack…if you don't drink, don't start.)

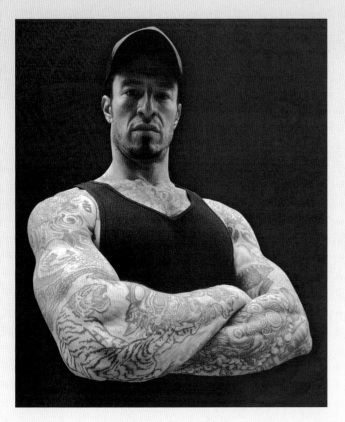

4. Stress hormones interfere with digestion. Relax after you eat. Listen to music. Watch shitty TV. Chill!

5. After a big meal, wait an hour before you train. Digestion re-routes a large volume of your blood supply to your gut. If it's in your belly, it can't get to your muscles. (This is why mom toldja to wait half an hour after eating before going swimming. She didn't want you drowning, moonbeam.)

6. You don't mention stress or sleep. Your new job for three months—getting ten SOLID hours of Zs per day. If you can't fit it in at night, learn to nap during the day.

7. *Believe.* There is a very real biology of faith. Start seeing yourself as alpha—for these four months—and it WILL happen.

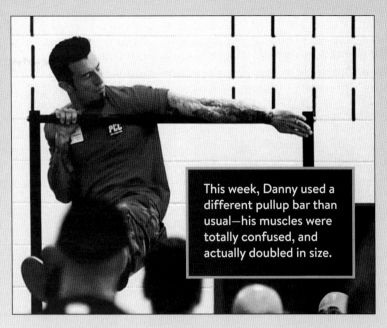

This week, Danny used a different pullup bar than usual—his muscles were totally confused, and actually doubled in size.

Q. I've read in several bodybuilding magazines that I need to change my exercises frequently in order to "confuse" my muscles into growth. Is that true?

A. Muscle cells are binary creations. They can only contract or relax. That's all they can do. If the muscle cells in your pectorals are firing, they don't know whether you are doing dips, pushups or work on the gymnastic rings. They have no idea. The idea that changing your exercises could "confuse" (or "shock") your muscle cells is absurd.

For sure, performing similar exercises over a long period can stress the joints or connective tissues from a certain angle, possibly causing stiffness or some post-workout aching. For this reason, it can be good to swap your exercises around from time to time. Of course, if you're carrying an injury, you might need to change your training routine entirely, to reflect that fact.

The real value of variety is in making your training *interesting*. The muscle cells can't get bored, but the mind sure can—and quickly. It's a great idea to alter your program a little every 6-8 weeks, just to keep things feeling fresh, fun and creative. The changes can be minor—a different rep range, workout order, a new finisher—but try to make *some* changes. Not for your muscles, but for your mind!

Q. I read in several bodybuilding magazines that I need to eat protein every 2-3 hours to have a hope in hell of growing. They also say that I need a huge amount of protein, like two grams per pound of bodyweight. Why don't your Commandments mention the need for protein?

A. I discussed the "protein myth" fully in *Convict Conditioning 2*. You do not require large, frequent doses of protein to reach the upper-level of your natural genetic potential. If you eat more protein than a healthy diet demands, that extra protein will not be turned into muscle. Muscle is *not* made up of protein, anyway—about 70% of muscle is water. If you drank extra gallons of water each day, do you think it would get turned into muscle, ballooning them arms up like Popeye? Nope—you'd just piss out the stuff your body didn't require. Extra protein can't be discarded so easily, so the body turns it into sugars and fats. As a result, a diet overloaded with protein is more likely to give you a huge gut than huge guns. In jail, I witnessed countless athletes build gigantic muscles on diets fairly low in protein. In fact, we had diets that would be considered laughably shitty by modern fitness standards.

If this is true—and it is—then why do all the magazines tell you to use such high levels of protein supplements? Simple. Because—universally—they are owned or sponsored by companies who manufacture and sell this worthless shit.

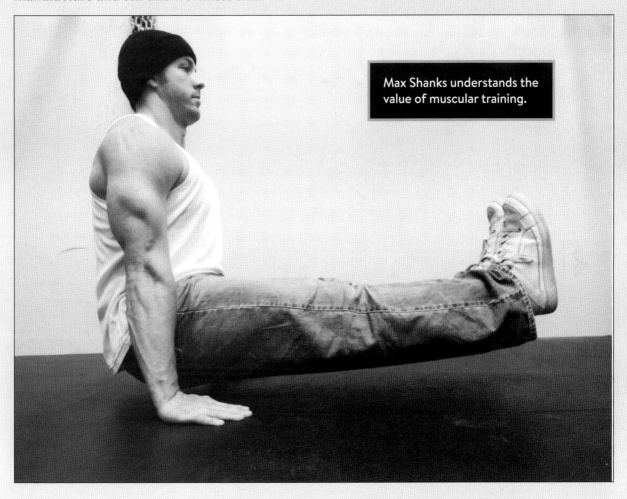

Max Shanks understands the value of muscular training.

Q. I have heard that whey is the "perfect" food for building muscle. Is this true?

A. It amazes me how many rubes have been taught to worship *whey*. Since the beginning of dairy farming, whey has been considered little more than a nasty by-product of cheese-making. (Blessed are the cheese-makers, huh? Bonus points if you actually get that reference.) When you make cheese (by either souring milk or adding rennet), dairy milk splits into two different compounds; *curds*, and *whey*.* (These are essentially two different types of proteins; everybody has heard of *whey* protein, but curds are better known to bodybuilders as *casein*.)

Curds are thick and tasty, and they are the stuff which is pressed into delicious, nutritious cheese—high in protein, calcium and healthy fats, and absorbed slowly by the body. Whey is the watery, unpleasant gunk which rises to the surface. For years, cheese-makers used to throw this crap away. They must have jumped for joy at the Cheese Marketing Board meeting when somebody finally found a use for it—dry it into a powder and sell it as an overpriced supplement to dummies who expect to mix it, drink it, and look like Hulk Hogan in six months! Bwah, ha ha!

The reason whey is supposedly so friggin' wonderful is pretty simple. It absorbs quickly into the bloodstream. Unfortunately, the human body builds muscle at an *incredibly* slow rate—and most of it's done during sleep—which means that a sudden spike in blood protein during the day is pretty useless. Actually, it's completely useless! Curds on the other hand, turn into a kind of *gel* when they hit the stomach. They "curdle" easily (hence the name *curds*). This means that the body absorbs curds easily and slowly over a longer period. It not only means you stay fuller longer, but that your body actually has more chance of actually assimilating some of the protein.

My opinion? Save your money on the whey and have a cheap, old-fashioned cheese sandwich instead. It's better muscle food!

*Remember the old nursery rhyme? Little Miss Muffet sat on her tuffet, eating her curds and whey. Well, that's where curds and whey come from. Don't ask me what the f*** a "tuffet" is, though. Maybe her ass, I don't know.

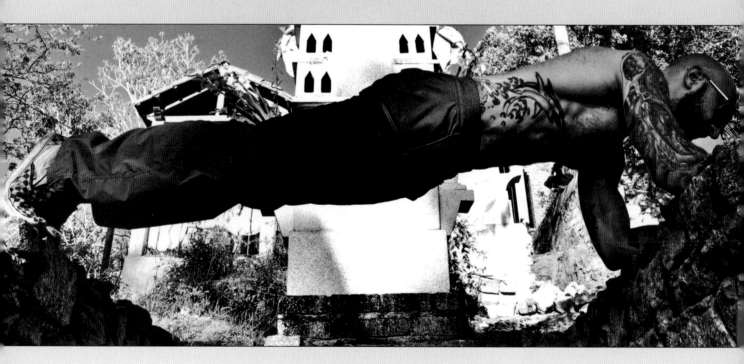

6

THE DEMOCRATIC ALTERNATIVE...

HOW TO GET AS POWERFUL AS POSSIBLE WITHOUT GAINING A POUND

I you are anything like me, you love *muscle*, and the idea of getting as big as you can. It motivates you to train. Men *should* look big and strong—don't we get told that since childhood? Hasn't every multi-colored comicbook panel taught us that as gospel since we first picked 'em up in our grubby, infantile paws?

So you might be thinking: *who the f*** would want to gain maximum strength without gaining any muscle with it? That's kinda like going to work and not bothering to pick up your paycheck at the end of the day, right?*

Wrong. There are a whole bunch of folks who either want (or need) massive strength and power, but without the attendant muscle bulk. Competitive athletes who compete in weight classes are one example; wrestlers, MMA athletes, boxers, etc. Females are another group who, as a rule, want to get stronger when they train, but without adding much (or any) size. Some men desire steely, whip-like power but see the sheer weight of mass as non-functional—many martial artists fall into this category; perhaps Bruce Lee was the archetype. Some guys just like to shock people by being relatively small and massively strong; Logan Christopher is a well-known bodyweight master and strongman who falls into this category.

Last but not least—bodybuilders also fall under this banner. Or, they should. As I pointed out in Commandment X of chapter 2, all athletes who want to become as huge as possible need to spend some portion of their time focusing on *pure strength*. Without a high (and increasing) level of strength, it's impossible to use enough load to stress your muscles into getting bigger. This is even truer once you get past a certain basic point.

Enough build-up. You want to build power like a Humvee, with the sleek lines of a classic Porsche? The following Ten Commandments got you covered, my boy. Follow them, and I promise you *cannot* fail, even if you had trouble getting stronger in the past. Your days of weakness are done, kid.

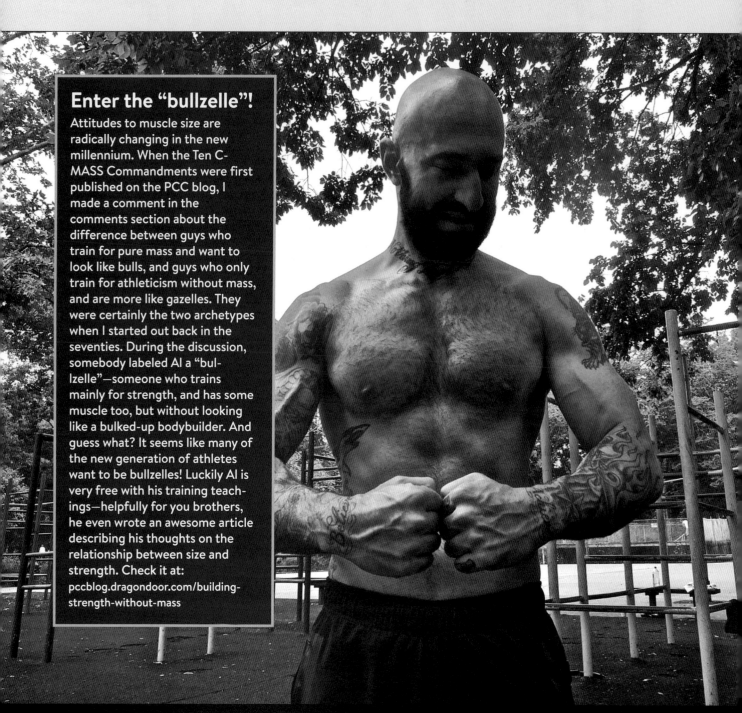

Enter the "bullzelle"!

Attitudes to muscle size are radically changing in the new millennium. When the Ten C-MASS Commandments were first published on the PCC blog, I made a comment in the comments section about the difference between guys who train for pure mass and want to look like bulls, and guys who only train for athleticism without mass, and are more like gazelles. They were certainly the two archetypes when I started out back in the seventies. During the discussion, somebody labeled Al a "bullzelle"—someone who trains mainly for strength, and has some muscle too, but without looking like a bulked-up bodybuilder. And guess what? It seems like many of the new generation of athletes want to be bullzelles! Luckily Al is very free with his training teachings—helpfully for you brothers, he even wrote an awesome article describing his thoughts on the relationship between size and strength. Check it at: pccblog.dragondoor.com/building-strength-without-mass

COMMANDMENT I: USE LOW REPS WHILE KEEPING "FRESH"!

When I was training in San Quentin, there was a saying:

> **"The first few reps are for strength, the last few reps are for muscle."**

What does this mean? Well, picture an average 8-rep set of pullups. You bodyweight is exactly the same for all eight reps, but during the first 1-3 reps your muscles are *crispest*; they possess the most contractile power. They are tensing the hardest. This is what strength really is—*the ability of the nervous system to elicit high-intensity contractions from the muscles*. So during these first reps you are training your strength.

During the last few reps, reps 6-8, your muscles are tired. They are no longer able to fire so hard—so you are not working your *nervous system* as powerfully as during reps 1-3. So these final reps are less efficient for strength training. But because you are depleting energy from the muscle cells, you are training your *muscles*, telling them they need to get bigger and swell with more chemical energy. This is what it means to say that the first reps are for strength (i.e., the nervous system) the last reps are for muscle.

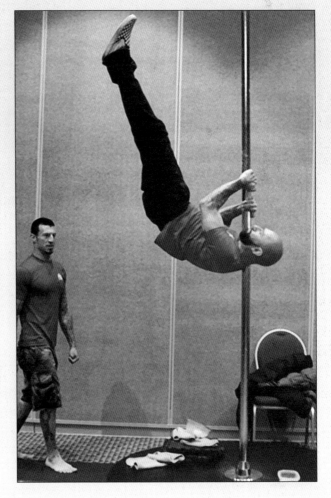

What does this mean in practice? Well, if you wanna generate huge strength without building muscle, pick an exercise you can perform maybe 6-8 reps *to failure* on. Then just do the first 3 reps...but do them as hard as you can, generating as much force, as much tension as you can. Then stop at rep 3...*even though you could do another 3-5 reps*. These days this is often called keeping "fresh" while you train. Keep the reps low, don't push to exhaustion, and take plenty of rest between sets.

This is the hard one for bodybuilders to get their noggins round. Athletes who want bigger muscles are used to really pushing their limits when they train; but this is actually a *bad* idea if you want peak strength with zero muscle gain.

Right about now, some of you wiseguys might be askin'; "why not just perform the 8-rep set? Wouldn't that give you strength (the first reps) AND size (the last reps)?" Well, you can. It's the basis of *Convict Conditioning*. However, this method will build strength and muscle together, and if *pure strength* is what you want, you should stay fresh.

Staying fresh also allows you to train *more often*—which leads us directly to Commandment II.

COMMANDMENT II: UTILIZE HEBB'S LAW—DRILL MOVEMENTS AS OFTEN AS POSSIBLE!

When bodybuilders train their muscles hard, those muscles adapt by building extra energy into the cells. They get bigger. This process can take a long time—days, and even *weeks* in some cases. This is why rest, nutrition and sleep are so sacred to bodybuilders. The growth happens during rest.

Pure strength training is different. Strength increases are largely due to the nervous system learning how to *communicate better* with the muscles. Imagine that the human biceps has a hundred muscle cells, each attached to a nerve (there are vastly more cells and I'm simplifying, but the basic picture is right). Muscle cells are binary—they don't fire "hard" or "soft"—they either contract completely or not at all. How much power you can squeeze outta that bicep depends mostly on *how many* of those muscle cells fire. The average human being can maybe get 25 of these cells to fire. But if they trained their nervous system to *communicate with their biceps better*, they might be able to get 75 of those cells to fire. Imagine that—tripling your strength, with no increase in muscle size! That—put basically—is how pure strength training works.

These two models are why *frequency*—how often you train—is often so radically different for pure strength trainers and for bodybuilders. Bodybuilders' muscles grow *when they rest*. A pure strength athlete's nervous system reconfigures *while they are training*.

The perfect bodybuilder would spend as *little time* training as possible—so they could spend more time growing. The perfect strength trainer would spend as *much time* training as possible—so their nervous system would reconfigure to the max.

Big brains out there call this *Hebb's Law,* named after the Canadian scientist (and honest-to-God genius) Dr Donald Hebb. Old Donald taught us that the nervous system adapts by forming new connections between nerve cells. How do we form these connections? *By repetition.* (Hebb's Law has been called "The Law of Repetition".)

You don't need to be a scientist to understand this law. We all learned as kids that the nervous system picks up new skills better if we practice more often—if we *drill.* It's how Bulgarian weight-lifters train their nervous systems to build strength, and it's how gymnasts—and acrobats, and martial artists—have trained to master bodyweight feats since the beginning of time. Training for *pure* strength and training to *master a skill* are virtually identical methods. They are both nervous system-based, and rely on Hebb's Law.

It's simple, boys and girls. As long as you keep fresh and keep your reps low (Commandment I), do as many sets as you can, as often as you can!

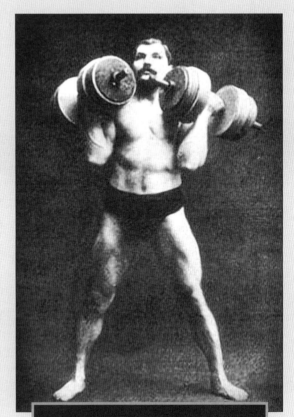

Arthur Saxon utilized Hebb's Law to become the strongest man on the planet. Never a very big athlete, he trained his nervous system by performing his trick lifts as often as possible, typically several times per day. You can do just the same with bodyweight—I call it *consolidation training* in **Convict Conditioning**.

PURE STRENGTH TACTICS:

- *Perform your most difficult movements as often as possible (without exhausting yourself)*

- *Use lots of sets, spaced over longer periods of time*

- *Drill, drill, drill!*

COMMANDMENT III:
MASTER MUSCLE SYNERGY!

Quick quiz, boys and girls: if you wanted to generate maximum force (that's what strength is, by the way), would it be easier to do with:

a. 10% of your muscles, or;
b. 100% of your muscles.

Simple huh? *Of course* the answer is *b*! All your muscles working *together* would be able to produce much more force than just a few of your muscles working *alone*.

If you wish to be strong, you need to teach your muscles to work in synergy with each other as well as is humanly possible. If there is a "secret" to being supremely strong, that's it in a nutshell. The knack of using your muscles all in a coordinated manner is one of the key features of a strength athlete—of any functional athlete, in fact. Look at an un-coordinated kid try and lift a weight above his head. He'll struggle and strain, and push with his arms and the tops of his shoulders. Now look at an Olympic weight-lifter do it. He's been trained to unlock the power of all his muscles in pushing a weight up—his legs, his midsection, his back, his chest—everything. *Boom*— the weight shoots up.

The same principle applies to bodyweight strength; you need to learn to use the force-generating capacity of all your muscles when you do a pushup—even your toes help a little! If the system ain't coordinated, it doesn't matter how big your individual muscles are, strength is not gonna happen.

This is one way in which strength training is very different from modern bodybuilding. Bodybuilders consciously *de-train* themselves of their athletic instinct to use their muscles in synergy. When doing curls, they deliberately turn off their shoulders and triceps—to place more stress directly on the biceps. When doing lateral raises, they deliberately relax and shut down their traps, their upper back, their legs and chest—so that all the pressure is applied to the side of the shoulders. Isolation is a sacred cow of modern bodybuilding.

If you want to get super-powerful, unlearn these ideas, which the magazines have no doubt thrown at you. Use exercises which require input from as many muscles as possible; try to use the big stuff which tests all your muscles to the max. I'm talking about:

• Kipping pullups
• Muscle-ups
• Pull-ups
• Pushups and dips
• Squats and pistols
• Rollovers, etc.

All of these exercises can be made progressive. Another great way to learn muscular coordination and control is to explore balancing exercises and static holds. These are typically fairly useless for bodybuilding, but because they encourage coordination and total-body tension they can radically enhance strength—gymnast style. Work with:

- Free handstands
- Bridges
- L-holds
- Front and rear hanging levers
- Elbow levers and planks
- Frog holds
- Human flags, etc.

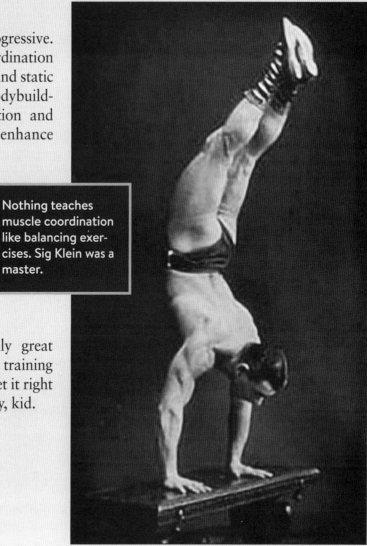

Nothing teaches muscle coordination like balancing exercises. Sig Klein was a master.

These techniques also work exceptionally great with the low rep, high volume/keep fresh training described in the previous Commandments. Get it right and pretty soon you'll be stronger than Spidey, kid.

COMMANDMENT IV: BRACE YOURSELF!

If there is a single tactic that's *guaranteed* to maximize your body-power in short order, it's *bracing*. Bracing—tensing the body—is both an art-form and a science. Bracing increases strength by a physiological phenomenon known as *irradiation*, whereby different branches of the nervous system are consciously "turned on" and primed for optimal performance.

Idea of bracing yourself is an ancient one, found in all Eastern martial arts. The most important thing to remember is that you can get better at it over time, if you practice and know the right "tricks". One trick, for example, is gripping the bar *hard* during pullups. This act of hard tension turns on neural pathways in the arms and lats, allowing you to pull harder than you could before. Bracing the abdominals correctly also increases strength—on just about any exercise—the Samurai with their *hara* training understood this perfectly. Pulling the shoulders tight into their

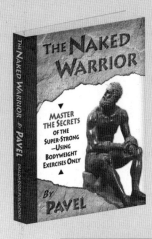

sockets activates the huge strength of the lats; even bracing the glutes can increase your squatting power, via irradiation. Brace!

When it comes to mastering bracing, there is only one man to go to for instruction—*Pavel Tsatsouline*. Pavel is the ultimate "guru" of this system of techniques, and his bodyweight book *The Naked Warrior* is a treasure chest of ideas to help you with bracing, and pure strength development generally. It's not just "highly recommended" by me—it's the best book there is on the subject, hands down! If you don't already own that sucker, go to *Dragondoor.com* and get your hands on it as soon as possible.

PURE STRENGTH TACTICS:

- *Learn to isometrically brace ALL your muscles as iron-hard as possible*
- *Grip the bar hard as you can during pullups*
- *"Grip" the floor with your fingers when doing pushups*
- *Pull your arms down firmly into their sockets, to activate the powerful lats*
- *Keeps your abs tight and braced during training*
- *Squeeze and tense your glutes for strength*

COMMANDMENT V: LEARN OLD-SCHOOL BREATH CONTROL!

You ever see a boxer work the heavy bag? Didja notice how they all seem to *hiss* through their teeth when they let go with a heavy punch? You might have also seen a martial artist exhale sharply—a "kiai"—as they simultaneously unleash a high-power strike.

These fighting athletes understand the ancient relationship between breath and strength. Despite what you might have heard about "ki" or "chi", there's really nothing magical or mystical about the process. A huge amount goes on during breathing—probably more than you think. *Dozens* of muscles can contribute to respiration! Not just the diaphragm, but the abdominal muscles, the *sternocleidomastoid*, the *scalar muscles* (running from the chest up the neck), the *obliques*, the internal and external *intercostals* which cover the ribcage, amongst others. Think about it—when you add these muscles together, they cover virtually all of the torso and trunk. *Of course* breathing is going to have an effect on your ability to move powerfully!

If there is an instant "trick" to increasing your strength, it's *learning the art of the breath*. As mentioned, martial artists and boxers get this. Weight-lifters and powerlifters get it. All the old-time strongmen devoted space on breathing techniques and systems in their books and courses—all of 'em. They got it, too.

A lot of trainers tell their rubes that their breathing during strength training will give them energy. (It increases oxygen, right?) In fact, this is crap. Sure, breathing plenty is very useful for increasing stamina— mebbe during those high reps squats or leg raises—but oxygen has no immediate positive effect on *strength*. Pure strength training is *anaerobic*—it does not rely on oxygen at all, but liberates energy sources already present in the muscles. Most Olympic 100 meter sprinters don't breathe *at all* during a race. It's just a distraction.

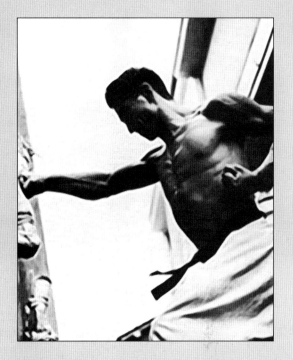

So why is inhalation—breathing in—so important for strength? The *PCC Instructor's Manual* sums it up in one shot:

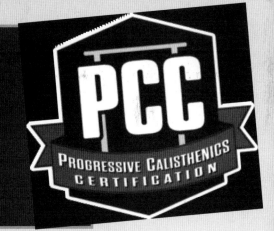

> *"Inhale to improve leverage. Breathing in a big lungful of air prior to a positive movement can increase strength on many techniques. When the lungs are full, pressure inside the trunk increases, making the torso more "solid" as a leverage base."*
>
> — From The PCC Instructor's Manual, page 537

The best time to inhale is prior to an eccentric (upwards) movement. Pushup experts understand this real well; full lungs can increase pressing strength by up to 10%, simply by altering the leverage of the ribcage. You *inhale* prior to the push, then *exhale* during the effort—ensuring that you time the exhalation to last as long as the movement (*slow hiss* for a strength move, *rapid puff* for explosives).

A controlled, forceful exhalation activates the muscles of the trunk, core and ribcage. These muscles, in combination, act as the axle, the central anchor for the extremities to exert voluntary force. The more braced, contracted and solid this structure is, the harder your limbs can push or pull. *The stronger the exhalation, the stronger the force production*—that's why fighters hiss or exhale that way when they punch or kick.

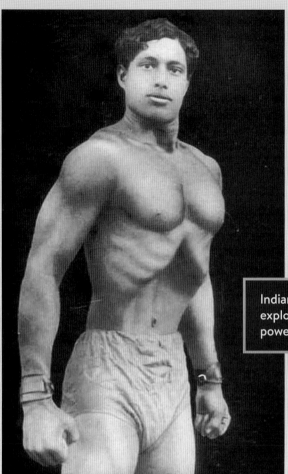

You can learn this too—it just takes practice. Oh yeah, and a bitchin' set of respiratory muscles—like titanium armor around your chest and lungs—don't hurt, either. Many convicts perform deliberate deep breathing exercises after their workout for just this reason—I still do this today. Relaxes you and oxygenates your blood, also. Win-win, disciple o' mine.

Indian muscle-control experts of the last century typically exploited yoga breathing methods to pack their torsos with power. (Model unknown, c.1930.)

PURE STRENGTH TACTICS:

- *Learn to inhale fully prior to a rep*
- *Exhale forcefully on the positive*
- *Practice deep breathing exercises to maximize your respiratory muscles and lungpower*

COMMANDMENT VI: TRAIN YOUR TENDONS!

When the old-time strongmen talked about strength, they rarely talked about muscle power—they typically focused on the integrity of the *tendons*. Check out this quote from one of the strongest of the old-school strongmen, "the Amazing Samson", Alexander Zass (b.1888):

> *"A large biceps is no more criterion of strength than a swollen abdomen is of digestion. It is the pulling tendon of the biceps that counts...some men with thin legs are stronger than some with thick legs. Why? Because strength lies in the tendons. Those unseen tough sinews which are the second in strength and density to the bones themselves. The tendons are the powerful fibrous attachments of the muscles to the bones. THEY ARE, IN SHORT, THE MASTER KEY TO THE STRENGTH WHICH OVERCOMES GREAT RESISTANCE. (Original emphasis)"*
>
> *— Alexander Zass from Samson's System and Methods, page 6*

Anyone who has pored over old-school strength literature (and you should, if you want to get as strong as possible) will recognize this training philosophy instantly. Different strongmen all had distinct methods for increasing tendon power and health, but they *all* included methods of tendon training as core aspects of their systems.

So how do you really train the tendons? The old timers believed in the concept of "supple strength". I talk in-depth about this in *Convict Conditioning 2*, but the basic concept is that *the tendons and connective tissues are best trained when stretched*. This is sometimes called *tension-flexibility*.

The old-school philosophy of building *supple strength* is the polar opposite of the modern approach. Modern bodybuilders typically have big muscles and weak joints. Just speak to the average bodybuilder who uses modern in-gym methods, and they will tell you that this is true—

they are always getting joint pain, injuries, etc. Hell, half the pros are addicted to painkillers for this very reason. This is because these men tend to focus on the top range of a motion, to work their muscles more. Look at folks on the leg press machine; inevitably, they are pumping out tiny reps with a huge weight.

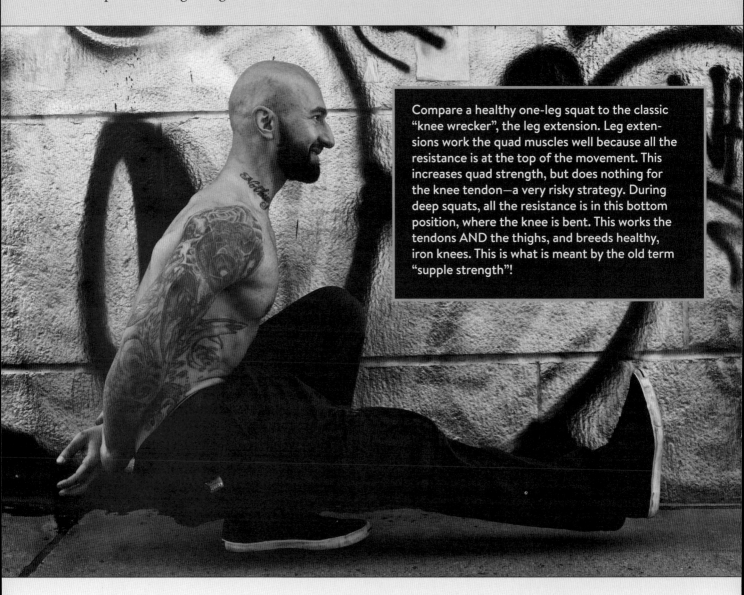

Compare a healthy one-leg squat to the classic "knee wrecker", the leg extension. Leg extensions work the quad muscles well because all the resistance is at the top of the movement. This increases quad strength, but does nothing for the knee tendon—a very risky strategy. During deep squats, all the resistance is in this bottom position, where the knee is bent. This works the tendons AND the thighs, and breeds healthy, iron knees. This is what is meant by the old term "supple strength"!

The exact same could be said of upper-body work. Most bodybuilders these days are in love with cable-type machines. Why? Because most of these movements encourage what bodybuilders call *peak contraction*. Peak contraction means that most of the force in the movement is at the top, with less at the bottom. This means that the muscles get plenty of benefit, but the tendons—which take the force at the bottom of the movement—get very little work. This approach pumps up the muscles, but weakens the tendons and joints over time. This leads to a lack of "real life" strength, as well as joint pain and injury. Of course, as an athlete's joints get sorer, they tend to avoid loading their tendons, and use the peak contraction-type techniques more and more. Many veteran lifters drop full movements altogether, and stick to partials in the top-range. And so the problem gets worse, until something pops for good.

One of the reasons calisthenics is good for real world strength is that—unlike machines, cables and bodybuilding-style techniques—it encourages the kind of full-range/loaded-under-tension movements which build supple strength and train the tendons. Basic movements like:

- Pullups
- Pushups
- Full squats

are meant to be practiced deep, and with the muscles stretched *while still loaded*. The more you stretch a muscle, the less it can contract; and this is why full, deep movements throw much of the load onto the tendons, making them stronger. The safest way to do this is as nature intended—bodyweight, baby!

PURE STRENGTH TACTICS:

- *Focus on the basic calisthenics moves*
- *Use exercises which safely load your tendons on the stretch*
- *Go as deep as you safely can on your exercises (without exaggerated motions)*
- *Hold your reps at the bottom for added benefit—never bounce*
- *Avoid machines or exercises which offer no resistance at the bottom of a rep*

COMMANDMENT VII:
FOCUS ON WEAK LINKS!

Big chest and shoulders! Huge back! Bulging quads! Bodybuilders want to gain as much mass as possible. The classical—and *best*—way to do this, is to focus all your attention on the biggest, strongest muscle groups...the legs, back, and chest. This is why all the time-tested get-big-quick programs feature exercises like deadlifts, rows, bench presses, and—especially—those beloved barbell squats (20-rep squat routines, milk 'n squats workouts, etc). Bodybuilding-based calisthenics programs similarly focus on the big muscles via dips, chins, one-leg squats, and so on.

For gaining weight as fast as your frame will allow, this makes some kinda sense. You pour all your energy into the largest muscle groups, to get the biggest bang for your bodybuilding buck.

Unfortunately when it comes to strength, this approach doesn't work as well. Any engineer will tell ya that the strength of a system ain't determined by it's biggest, *strongest* areas—it's determined by its *weakest* areas. The same goes for a human athlete. You are only as strong as your weakest link.

For this reason, if you want to maximize your strength potential, don't limit yourself to the exercises which focus on the biggest muscle groups. You also need to pay attention—extra attention—to the weakest areas. These include:

- **Grip:** hanging work, finger holds, fingertip pushups, towel hangs
- **Gut:** leg raises, rollovers, L-holds
- **Waist and spine:** bridges, planks, levers
- **Lateral chain:** twisting movements, flags, etc.

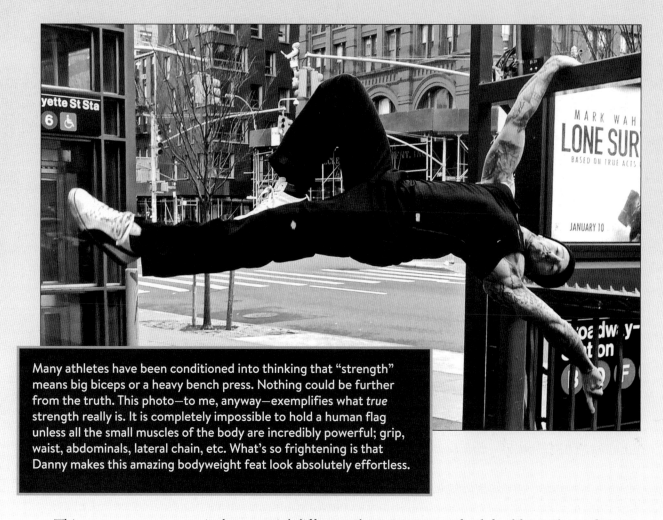

Many athletes have been conditioned into thinking that "strength" means big biceps or a heavy bench press. Nothing could be further from the truth. This photo—to me, anyway—exemplifies what *true* strength really is. It is completely impossible to hold a human flag unless all the small muscles of the body are incredibly powerful; grip, waist, abdominals, lateral chain, etc. What's so frightening is that Danny makes this amazing bodyweight feat look absolutely effortless.

This—to me, anyways—is the essential difference between a mere *bodybuilder* and a *truly powerful* human being. Size is not the issue. The issue is whether the small, invisible muscles are toughened as well as (or *better* than) the big, showy muscles. The Mighty Atom did it, Bruce Lee did it, Logan Christopher does it, and it worked out pretty well for them, huh?

COMMANDMENT VIII: EXPLOIT NEURAL FACILITATION!

We are talking about training the nervous system here, right? Well, the nervous system—like most sophisticated biological systems—possesses different sets of *gears*. If you ask the average dude to clench his arm muscles as tight as he can, he could probably not clench them all that hard; a mild tension, not much else. His arm nerves go from neutral to maybe first, second gear.

Compare this to the same dude holding a telephone when a bolt of lightning hits the line. Some people hit by lightning tense their arms with such unbelievable force that their clenching muscles literally *snap their bones in half*. It's not the electricity that does this—it's just the person's own muscles. The electricity just bypasses the brain and tells the nervous system to instantly shoot into top gear. The hidden reserves of nervous strength this reveals is very, very telling.

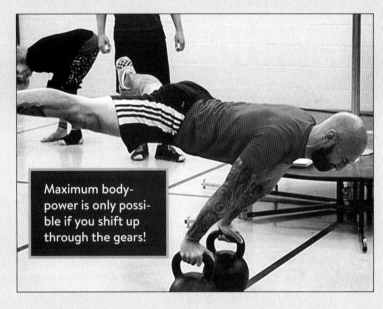

Maximum body-power is only possible if you shift up through the gears!

In everyday life, we can't suddenly tap into this power, the ability to shift our nervous system to the max gear. The brain has a dampener circuit, preventing it. The reason why is probably obvious—if we did it, we'd be constantly injuring ourselves; remember the arm bones snapping in half? Yikes!

There is, however, a pretty simple method of reaching the highest gear your brain will allow you to access. It's called *neural facilitation*—also known as *warming up*. Over time you can request your brain to release more and more neural energy to your muscles. The process begins in seconds, but can take minutes. If you ever go to a powerlifting meet, this is why guys are allowed to get under the bar and do reps before their main attempts—it's not to prevent *injury*, it's to make them *stronger*. There's not a healthy human being alive who is at their strongest on the first rep of an exercise—you need to build into it to truly reach your max for the day.

For example, virtually no strong guys would just up and attempt a one-arm pullup. It's simply too tough—most people would fail, because their nervous systems aren't releasing enough energy to achieve this. Their arms and lats are still in first gear. But if you did a couple easy reps of pullups (second gear), then rested, then did a couple reps of close pullups (third gear), then rested, then did an easy rep of an assisted one-arm (fourth gear), guess what—you could probably then try the one-arm and achieve it. The movement would seem easier because of neural facilitation; you woke up your nervous system and hit fifth gear!

The above is just an example. It may not match your strength range, but whatever your relative strength, the principle holds true—if you spend a few minutes working into your hardest exercises, you will wind up much stronger than if you didn't.

COMMANDMENT IX: APPLY PLYOMETRIC PATTERNS TO HACK NEURAL INHIBITION
(A.K.A. "MOVE FAST SOMETIMES"!)

Internet conversations—on a forum, in online comments and whatnot—are governed by something called *Godwin's Law*. This law states that: *As an online discussion grows longer, the probability of a comparison involving Nazis or Hitler approaches 1*. In other words, it's gonna happen.

These days, there's definitely something similar going on with strength—something you didn't see twenty, fifteen, or even ten years back in conversations about strength. But today—and definitely online—if two dudes are having a conversation about strength, then real quick, one of them will try to use the word *tension*. It's the big buzzword when it comes to strength in the modern era.

In a sense, that's good. But in another sense, it's kinda limiting. To most athletes, tension means contracting your muscles—all your inter-related muscles—as hard as you can. Sure, this is *bracing*,

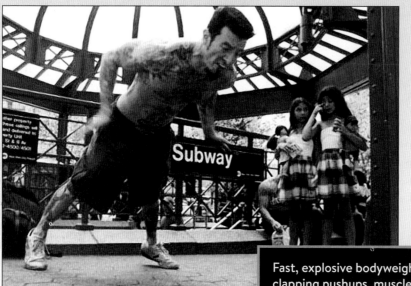

and it means rock hard, stable, brawn. But it also means *tightness*. And—worst of all—*slowness*. Most folks associate high-tension with very slow movements, or isometrics. It is impossible to move rapidly when your muscles remain tense. And this is fatal to a bodyweight master; as you develop, you should learn to move slow *and* fast.

Fast, explosive bodyweight movements—like clapping pushups, muscle-ups, flips and jumps—all bypass the brain's neural inhibition reflex. Nature's own little strength hack!

In fact calisthenics athletes have long understood that very fast movements—called "plyometrics" these days—can hugely increase strength. Think of your muscle cells as little light bulbs; the more bulbs that fire, the more light is given off. During high-tension static holds—or negatives, like a negative one-leg squat—your leg muscles light up like torches, as the nerves tell a certain amount of muscle cells to fire to keep you tense.

Next, imagine the same athlete performing a super-fast movement—jumping off a box, and immediately rebounding back up again. What happens to the leg muscles? No longer beaming out like slow torches, they go off for a fraction of a second like a high-power camera flash!

Why the radical output? When we perform slow, deliberate movements—no matter how tense we make ourselves—the nervous system limits the amount of muscle cells you can access, just to be on the safe side. It dampens the electrics, dials down the machine to prevent overkill. This is what smartasses call *neural inhibition*. You got no say in this kid. It's an automatic cerebral reflex which occurs on a totally subconscious level.

There is a *hack*, though. However, when your muscles are forced to move fast—like when you jump down or up, or during explosive bodyweight movements off the floor or the bar—then this dampening inhibition gets turned off. This makes perfect sense—you don't need maximum muscle power when performing voluntary, slow actions. Your body says *no*. But when you are forced to perform high-velocity *reactions* to gravity and your environment, your body adapts to the emergency and gives you the keys to the Humvee.

The take-home is simple. Sure, work with high-tension, slow stuff to build your voluntary strength. But to really get an edge, amp up your nervous strength, and reinforce those maximum-power neural patterns your bod is capable of, to perform *explosive* bodyweight work as part of your program.

How do you do this? Plyometric bodyweight work. As to the details, I've answered all the questions in **Convict Conditioning 3**. CC 3 will be to *explosive power* and *neurological fitness,* what **Convict Conditioning** was to *slow-strength* and *muscle gain.*

Like the first book, it's going to be a game-changer. Grab a copy in 2015.

COMMANDMENT X: MASTER THE POWER OF THE MIND!

If there is one drug that scares the shit out of American cops, it's PCP; phencyclidine, also known as *KJ*, *angel dust* and—tellingly—*amp*. The effects of PCP are the stuff of legend. While on PCP, police have recorded cases of men who:

- Have snapped steel handcuffs (in front of their bodies AND behind their backs)
- Taken on ten cops at once and held their own
- Kicked open locked police car doors from the inside
- Shrugged off bullet wounds at point blank range, and kept coming

Can you see now why cops shudder at the thought of PCP? Compared to amp, steroids ain't shit! Essentially, PCP turns average skinny bitches into goddam superheroes. (Until they wake up the next day; in which case, their bodies may be permanently crippled. If they wake up at all.)

Now, here's the interesting thing. PCP is not a steroid, or a performance enhancing drug, as we would understand the term. It does virtually nothing to the body at all to account for these incredible effects. Pencyclidine is a psychiatric drug. It is a powerful hallucinogenic—it's effects are mainly on the *mind*. The drug is able to put normal—often de-motivated—minds into such a high, psychotic state of arousal and emotion, that the body is forced to respond to supernormal levels.

Now, don't be an idiot. *Of course* I'm not suggesting you should take PCP before training. Not if you want to keep your f***ing teeth, anyhow. But the examples should make a point—that the mind really can make the body achieve incredible levels of strength and ferocity, even in relatively small, untrained guys. If the mind has this power on PCP, *it must also possess the same power without such drugs.*

So how do we harness that power? I could write a book on this topic, but for now I'm gonna hand

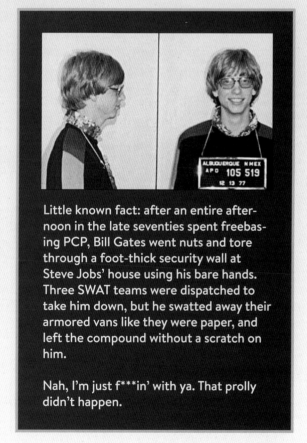

Little known fact: after an entire afternoon in the late seventies spent freebasing PCP, Bill Gates went nuts and tore through a foot-thick security wall at Steve Jobs' house using his bare hands. Three SWAT teams were dispatched to take him down, but he swatted away their armored vans like they were paper, and left the compound without a scratch on him.

Nah, I'm just f***in' with ya. That prolly didn't happen.

you the fundamentals you need to explore if you want to take your mental training to the next level, and optimize your strength:

1. AROUSAL

When the mind is amped up or "psyched", the body releases endorphins and adrenaline, which remove pain and increase power. If you can get into a controlled frenzy before a max attempt, you can radically increase your strength.

2. BELIEF

If you don't believe you can perform a bodyweight feat, your body is unlikely to disagree with you. But if you believe—if you *know*—you have the strength to do something, the sky is the limit. The record books are crammed with examples of this.

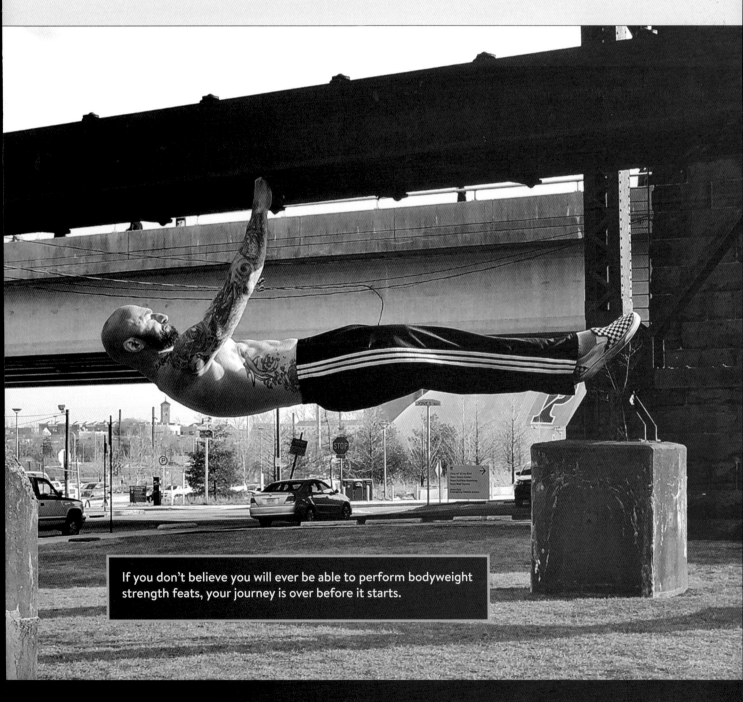

If you don't believe you will ever be able to perform bodyweight strength feats, your journey is over before it starts.

3. VISUALIZATION

This is linked to belief. Numerous studies show that the simple act of visualizing yourself doing something difficult makes you more likely to achieve it. Why? The brain is full of safety blocks and dampeners which limit our performance. When the brain "sees" us safely achieving something—even if the image is fake—it happily turns off some of those blocks.

4. MOTIVATION

Imagine going to train and finding that you are too weak to perform your usual handstand pushups. Suddenly a gangbanger enters the room, holding a gun to the head of the person you love most in the world—threatening to kill them if you can't do the exercise. Guess what—you'd get ten reps! Many athletes put themselves in fantasy situations before a tough set; maybe you'll win a million bucks for each rep, save the world or screw the girl?

5. IMAGINATION

At the heart of all these techniques is *imagination*. To achieve great strength you don't need *toughness* or *willpower* as much as *imagination*. An athlete with a powerful imagination can achieve wonderful things. All true legends began as fantasists, who dreamt about what they wanted to achieve, years before they ever got there. Imagination is underrated—it ain't just for kids. Cherish yours. Value it, use it, and it will grow stronger!

Trust me, these techniques can help you, but they are only the very surface. These days, we focus so much on the superficial aspects of physical culture—buff muscles, a nice tan, good teeth—that we ignore the most important, deeper currents. Throughout history there have been astonishing examples of men and women who have performed phenomenal physical feats, all through tapping into their mind's innate power. Tibetan monks can meditate in freezing wastes, and generate enough heat to melt icy sheets placed over their naked torsos. Yogis can control their heart-rate to such a degree that they can virtually stop it from beating. Soldiers so badly injured they should be dead have summoned the endurance not only to live, but to drag their comrades out of danger on the battlefield. The mind is amazing.

Can you imagine what you could do if you could explore your own mind and tap into just a tiny percentage of that inner force, to apply it to your bodyweight training? You could achieve miracles!

I believe in you, kid. You might think I'm lying, but I really, really do. If you are reading this, I'm pulling for you more than you know.

Now go do great things!

To recap, here are all Ten "Pure Strength" Commandments, lassoed and rounded up:

THE 10 COMMANDMENTS OF MASS-FREE STRENGTH

I: Use Low Reps While Keeping "Fresh"!

II: Utilize Hebb's Law—Drill Movements as Often as Possible!

III: Master Muscle Synergy!

IV: Brace Yourself!

V: Learn Old-School Breath Control!

VI: Train Your Tendons!

VII: Focus on Weak Links!

VIII: Exploit Neural Facilitation!

IX: Apply Plyometric Patterns to Hack Neural Inhibition!

X: Master the Power of the Mind!

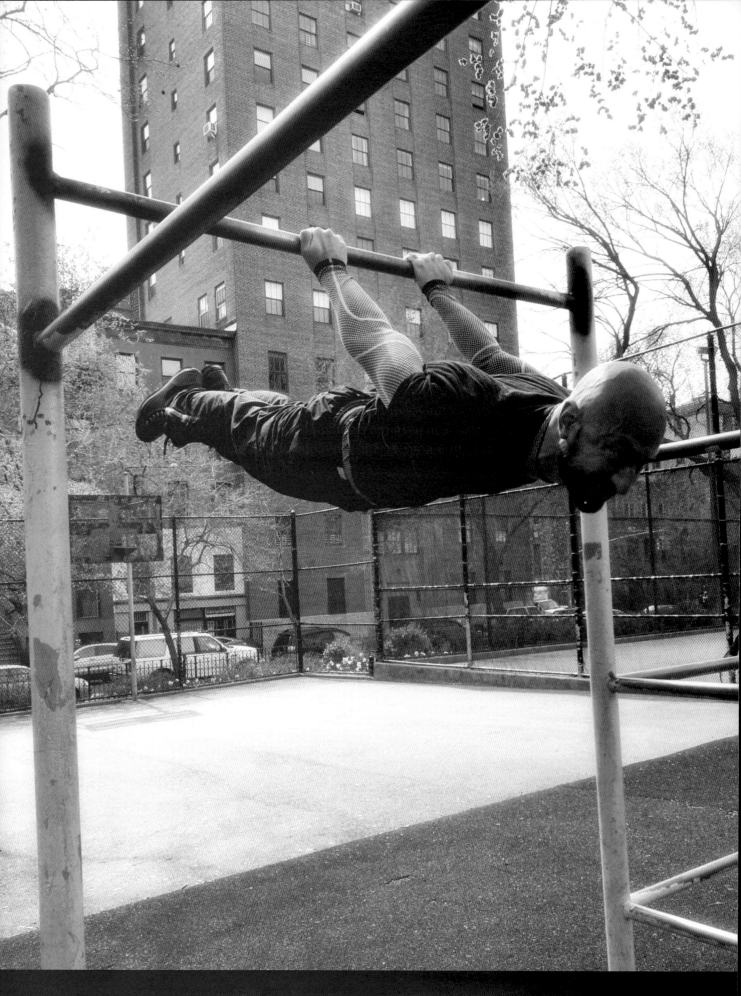

C-MASS — CALISTHENICS MASS

BONUS CHAPTER:

7

SUPERCHARGING YOUR HORMONAL PROFILE

This little book is, in all likelihood, the last word I will ever put out on bodyweight bodybuilding. So I'm going to devote my final thoughts on the matter to an aspect of muscle-building that's real close to my heart.

My ultimate message to all of you reading is this: *please don't take steroids.*

Ever. You don't need them, and they will only work against you in the long run. And I'm about to tell you why, homeboy.

HORMONES AND MUSCLE GROWTH

Truth time. I have devoted my life to training others, and writing about training. But your *hormones* are what build muscle. All the training is pretty secondary. *Getting a tan* is a great analogy for building muscle. Let's say the amount of time you spend sunbathing is like your bodybuilding training. The strength of the sun is like your hormonal level.

Let's face it, you can lie in the sun all goddam day, but if the sun is weak—say, you live in the north of Scotland in winter—you ain't gonna get a tan. It's unlikely your skin will change much at all. But if you live in Dubai, you only need to take your shirt off for a couple minutes and your skin will begin to change and adapt.

Muscle-building is exactly the same. You can work out hard as possible as often as possible, but if your hormonal levels aren't good, your gains will be close to nil. You can see this for yourself in the real world. The average guy can go to the gym and work hard and build some meat on himself. But if his girlfriend goes to the same gym and tries just as hard, the chances of her building any significant muscle are almost zip. They can eat the same, train the same, rest the same and have the same mindset. What's the difference? Hormonal levels. Men, in general, have about ten times more testosterone than girlies.

A woman training hard on tough calisthenics exercises will become stronger and more "toned" (yeah, I hate the word too), but she won't ever become muscular. She cannot. Ever watch the Olympics? Often the most powerful female gymnasts on the planet—provided they are drug-free—really don't look much bigger

Adrienne Harvey is a Senior PCC and a phenomenal bodyweight athlete. Beautiful, elegant and strong, but she is never going to be mistaken for a big bodybuilder!

than the average in-shape female. They certainly don't look like *bodybuilders*. This is true even though they are many, many times proportionately stronger than the average male slob.

As soon as we grasp the true role of hormones—in particular, *testosterone*—in muscle-building, it becomes clear that our training methods are, in fact, kinda secondary. If you want to get big and strong—and stay big and strong over an extended lifetime—your primary concern should be building up your test levels. Studies and simple experience have demonstrated that, far from being some esoteric practice, this is completely achievable—some men have increased their diminished total testosterone levels by *over a thousand percent!* How? Just by following a few basic rules.

What rules? Listen up, Boy Wonder. This is the most important bodybuilding advice anyone will ever give you.

THE 6 RULES OF TESTOSTERONE BUILDING

Here are the basic rules to follow if you want to build up your testosterone levels. Some experts list dozens of ways to jack up your testosterone—often these methods include vitamin supplementation. This is all great for the supplement companies, but the reality is that unless your vitamin levels (zinc, for example) are dangerously low, your hormonal production won't suffer; in other words, studies show that extra vitamins don't actually increase your testosterone levels one damn bit, as long as you eat a fairly balanced diet in the first place.

Over the years I've heard various bizarre suggestions to increase test, from spanking the monkey, to handling a powerful gun (the same thing, in my case). In truth, testosterone can spike or dip slightly for various reasons, most of which are superficial and temporary. The following rules are the most powerful and long-lasting, however. Follow them if you want to get diesel.

RULE 1: TRAIN HARD

A lot of ink has been spilt over exactly *why* and *how* hard physical work stimulates increases in testosterone, but very few experts now dispute that it does exactly that. To anybody who understands adaptation, it makes perfect sense. Your body runs on the biological principle of *homeostasis*. One way of putting homeostasis is to say that to save energy your body will *only ever do the minimum of what it has to do*. It wants an easy life. Testosterone is a powerful compound, evolved to build lean muscle. If your body thinks you survive by playing video games on the couch and eating Ding Dongs all day, why should your bod waste energy producing a surplus of test? You don't need it, right?

On the other hand, if you have to *struggle* to survive—and grinding through hard pushups, pullups and other exercises seems like a struggle to your body—then your body adapts by manufacturing powerful testosterone, so you can build the tools to get the job done and make life easier. Your body is smart, but it only responds to the signals you give it.

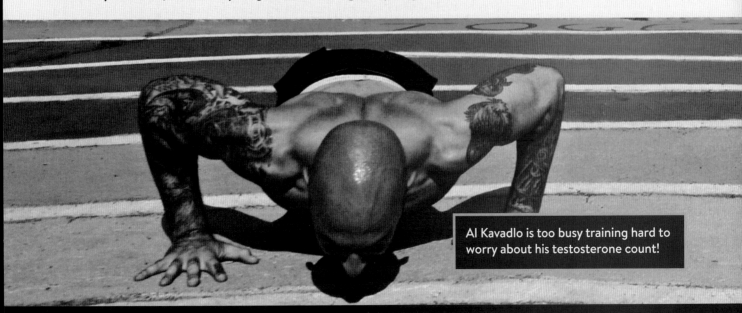

Al Kavadlo is too busy training hard to worry about his testosterone count!

RULE 2: SLEEP LONG AND DEEP

This issue is so serious, I made it one of my C-MASS commandments in chapter 2. Most growth—whether it's an iceberg, or a plant, or a human being—takes place in the *darkness*. Bodybuilding is like this. Very few bodybuilders realize that testosterone is only generated by your balls *at night*. More specifically, test production peaks during the REM (*Rapid Eye Movement*) phase of sleep (as a rule of thumb, this is when you are dreaming). The key thing to remember here is that there are relatively few REM phases during the first several hours of sleep; but the longer you doze, the more REM sleep you get until your sleep is nearly full of it. Long story short: every minute more you sleep, the more testosterone your body will pump out for you.

Most human beings in America (with the exception of prison inmates) are chronically sleep deprived. The general advice of 6-8 hours is WAY too low in my opinion. How much is "too much"? Unless you have a brain tumor, there is no "too much" for a bodybuilder. If you can get away with sleeping fourteen hours a day, f***ing do it. Some folks will say that's "antisocial". Compared to what? Staying awake and whacking off while playing Xbox?

RULE 3: DON'T BE A BIG FAT FATTY

When tested, morbidly obese men are typically found to have through-the-floor testosterone levels. This is true whether they workout or not. This is gonna sound sexist (as always) but women are *meant* to have more bodyfat than males for purposes of childbirth. (Guys, you already intuitively understand this—at least your body does. When you are checking out a chick's tits or ass, you are really just looking at sexy fat storage.) For this reason, fat supplies in the body are inextricably associated with *estrogen,* the crazy-evil female hormone and the arch nemesis of our hero, testosterone.

Fat is often thought of as a passive tissue, but in fact fat cells are like little chemical factories. In particular, adipose (fat) cells generate *aromatase*, an enzyme which finds circulating testosterone (*muscles, strength*) and converts it into estrogen (*titties, crying over sunsets*). This is exactly why fat dudes have low testosterone. Every pound of lard is like an enemy base destroying the good stuff and replacing it with girl hormones. F***!

On the downside, this is a vicious cycle. The fatter you get, the less test you have, and the harder it is to build the muscle and lose the flab. The upside is the exact reverse of the downside...the more you grit your teeth and train, and avoid overfeeding, the more lard will melt from your body. With every pound lost, you gain a little more testosterone back, which makes further muscle gain and fat loss easier. See? Your body knows what to do. You just gotta *tell it*, kid.

RULE 4: CONSUME CHOLESTEROL

How do you make a hormone? ...Don't pay the bitch!

Yeah, it's an old, sexist joke. I'm, an old sexist, so it kinda makes sense. Seriously though, I discussed this in chapter 2 of this book. Essentially, what the low-fat bodybuilding brigade have forgotten is that testosterone is built from *cholesterol*—cholesterol forms the building blocks for test. That's why (drug-free) vegans typically have the muscle mass of a Ray Harryhausen walking skeleton. As long as you follow rule 1 and give your body enough hard exercise, and you follow rule 3 and don't allow yourself to become a lard-ass, cholesterol-based grub like eggs, sausage, cheese and fatty meat won't do you any harm. But it *will* increase your testosterone levels.

Cholesterol (*left*) is the main precursor of testosterone (*right*). Notice the similarity?

RULE 5: GO STRAIGHT EDGE

The philosophy of *straight edge* is something I talk about in *Convict Conditioning 2*. I could just as easily say: *don't smoke, don't drink, don't do drugs.*

I'm not trying to give you some kind of sermon here—this is just biology, bro. Smoking introduces carbon monoxide into the blood, and this chemical screws badly with your body's ability to convert cholesterol into testosterone. Alcohol reduces your test in several ways. Beer, for example, contains hops, which are a super-powerful phytoestrogen (i.e., a plant estrogen). Hops convert to estrogen so easily in the body that brewers discovered centuries ago that the women who harvested the hops had longer periods. It has always been understood that booze kills male sex drive—hence the term "brewer's droop". Interestingly, Protestants were behind the German *Beer Purity Law* during the Renaissance, because they understood that alcohol destroys the libido.

Another fact many athletes just haven't been told is that one of the jobs of the liver is to produce enzymes which limit the amount of estrogen in the body. When you take drugs (even over-the-counter meds) you f*** up your liver, and it can't limit the estrogen as well. One of the major signs of liver damage in male drug addicts and alcoholics is the presence of shrunken testicles and gynaecomastia— literally, titty growth. With so much estrogen in their bodies, their testosterone levels collapse.

Those five are the most important rules you can follow to improve your hormonal profile—in that order. But there is a sixth rule:

RULE 6: DON'T TAKE STEROIDS

I'll say it plain; *the most damaging thing a modern athlete can do to his hormonal profile is to take steroids.*

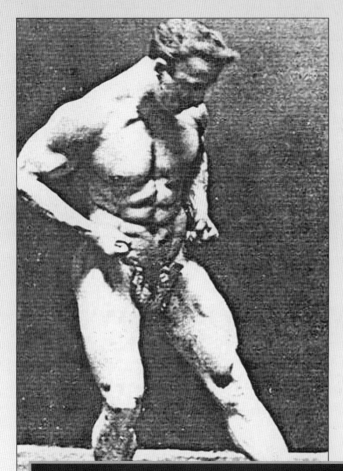

It is a modern myth that you need steroids and heavy weights to build an incredible physique. The above shot is of early bodybuilder Bobby Pandour. Pandour was born in 1876—testosterone wasn't syntheisized (from cholesterol!) until 1935, so this is one of the very few phenoms you can be sure was truly 100% natural. Pandour built his muscle exclusively using bodyweight training and muscle control (isometrics). He was convinced that lifting heavy external weights was bad for the body, and never lifted more than a 10lbs dumbbell in training! But he was as strong as hell, and had a physique that would blow many modern day steroid junkies out of the water. It can be done.

How can that be? A lot of folks will ask. Guys who take steroids put on tons of muscle, don't they? Well yeah, they *do*. But at a terrible price to their own, endogenous testosterone levels.

Like I said above, testosterone is basically what builds muscle. For this reason, all modern steroids are, essentially, synthetic versions of testosterone. From the moment you put these chemicals into your body, the principle of *homeostasis* takes over; your body figures that with all this "new" testosterone floating around, it doesn't need to make its own. So your own hormonal system begins shutting down—it literally commits suicide. This is howcome even moderate steroid users have shrunken balls—their testosterone factories (the *testes*) just shut down. This is why, over time, steroid users are plagued by "bitch tits"—gynaecomastia, a.k.a. breast production. This is incredibly common as bodybuilding today. That's right—all these big, strong bodybuilders are growing f***ing tits, like a Barbie doll!

Perhaps the worst part of this is that the damage is permanent. Yes, if you only take steroids for a short while you can often build your own testosterone back up to some degree—after many miserable months—but the longer you take, and the heavier the dose, the more permanent this damage to your hormonal system becomes. What you might not know is that long-term users *never* come off testosterone. They can't—their own bodies just don't make any anymore. Once they have damaged their hormonal system to a certain point, it can *never* recover. These men are totally dependent on their drugs, no different to an ill person being dependent upon dialysis. How is that strength? Remember, the whole point of bodybuilding is to build up your hormonal levels. By taking steroids, you are doing the exact opposite...you are destroying your body's own hormonal systems from the inside, out.

Despite what you might think, the medical industry are *pissed as hell* that steroids have been made illegal—because it means they can't peddle that vile shit for huge profits. They are getting round the law now, though. They are simply calling steroids "Testosterone Replacement Therapy" (TRT) and are selling the idea that modern men *need* steroids as *medicine* because we are all somehow "sick", and low in test. *This is just lies.* Modern men *are* low in

This is the latest method of TRT—find a huge gauge needle and inject bulky testosterone pellets into someone's ass. Hell, it works for cattle, right? Trouble is, these things often cause bleeding, nasty infections, or they simply fall out, rejected by the body (which clearly has more sense than its goddam owner).

test, but not because they are sick—it's because of their lifestyle. That's all. (I talk more about this modern myth of "low testosterone" in the next section.) I'm not demonizing steroids as medicine, by the way; there *really are* good medical reasons for taking steroids—such as to combat AIDS and fatal wasting diseases. Being a fat, lazy f***er is not a good reason, however.

Anybody who tells you that TRT "is not the same as steroids" is a f***ing retard who has allowed themselves to be fooled by pharmaceutical corporations. The drug delivery may be slightly different (and then again, it may not), but the substance is *fundamentally identical*. TRT is a modern confidence trick, designed to take your money and weaken your hormonal system. Why would "doctors" want to permanently weaken your natural testosterone levels? So they can keep selling you this shit your whole life!

Don't be under any illusions when you mess with exogenous hormones. This damage to your own hormonal system begins right away—from your first injection, from the first pill you put into your mouth. If you want to be strong and muscular into your old age, you can do it by following the rules I've given you, but if you take steroids, forget it. The modern steroid boom is a medical catastrophe waiting to happen. In a few years time, all these kids taking gear to look "buff" in the club are going to be in their forties, their fifties, with the test levels of an eighty year old grandmother.

Don't become one of these people. Dedicate your life to hard training and clean living, and you can be strong, muscular and healthy well into your old age—just like my mentor, Joe Hartigan who was busting out one-arm pullups in his *seventies*; just like Joe Greenstein, the "Mighty Atom", who was bending steel in his *eighties*; just like Manohar Aich, who was competing in bodybuilding contests in his *nineties*. They could do this because they followed the six simple rules in this chapter.

You can be like these great men. These six rules will increase your test levels significantly, in a matter of days. If you loyally follow these rules over months and years, you can radically build up your hormonal system over time, just like a bodybuilder painstakingly builds up his muscular system. The old-timers had more test in their *old age* than the average twenty-something desk jockey does *right now*. This is how they did it, and you can, also. Make it happen, brother!

THE MODERN TESTOSTERONE MYTH

Before I finish I want to take on one increasingly popular defense for steroids and TRT. This argument goes as follows:

> *Modern men live in a world full of environmental pollutants and toxins, and are forced to eat food which has been stripped of its nutrition due to industrial agriculture and food processing. For these reasons, it's impossible for the average man of today to possess normal levels of testosterone, like previous generations of males did.*

Guess what I say to this? *It's flat out nonsense!* In fact, it stinks worse than a hobo's cock cheese.

If athletes choose to take steroids, that's their business. But this argument is totally full of shit— it's a justification many lazy athletes have jumped all over though, and as a result I'm sure you've heard this horse-crap somewhere. Even athletes who consider themselves "old school" or "Spartan" admit to using testosterone, because they have bought into this shit! These weak-willed pricks wouldn't know old school if it kicked them in the ass.

For what it's worth, I got no doubt that as time goes by male testosterone levels *are* dropping. No *doubt at all*. In fact, I think the current generation is pretty much *testosterone-starved*. I just have to walk the streets and see these lazy-ass, Xbox playing, metrosexual, Justin Beiber-looking motherf***ers strutting all over to realize that. My problem is not with the suggestion that men have lower test levels than their forefathers did, my problem is with the theory as to *why*.

It's pretty obvious to anyone with a brain that as time goes on, men break the first five basic rules I gave above. This is increasingly true the more time goes by. *That's why testosterone is dropping*. Think about this:

- Our ancestors worked hard manual labor jobs with their hands—they got the equivalent of a tough workout every damn day. These days, more and more guys let machines do the work, or they sit behind desks. That's why their bodies aren't producing enough testosterone.

- Due to extended working patterns, we all sleep less now. Before the electric light was invented, most humans slept 10 or more hours a night…now the average worker gets 5-7 hours. Modern men just aren't getting the REM sleep they need to generate enough hormones.

- Obesity—which literally turns testosterone into estrogen—was so rare a hundred years ago, that fat people were exhibited as freaks in travelling shows. Now it's epidemic; it's almost the norm.

- Whereas previous generations thrived on fresh, healthy, high cholesterol food—eggs, ham, cheese, whole milk, lard—modern schlubs make do with highly processed, high-carb bullshit. And so the cycle deepens.

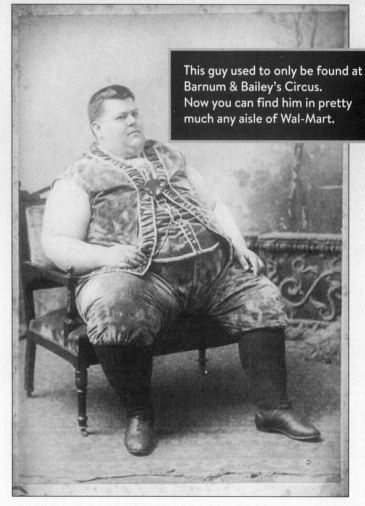

This guy used to only be found at Barnum & Bailey's Circus. Now you can find him in pretty much any aisle of Wal-Mart.

- Recreational drug and alcohol use has always existed, but it's much, much more prevalent in the modern USA than in previous years. This all chips away at testosterone.

…Am I right? Jesus, it's a wonder modern men have any testosterone at all!

This is exactly why men have less testosterone these days. It's got *jack shit* to do with this limp-green bullshit that the environment is all f***ed up and full of toxins and pollutants. For those of you concerned with modern toxins, I say this: *don't be such a f**ing pussy.* Jesus, cowering in the corner, quivering over every little chemical in the air and the food chain? No wonder your testosterone is low, you'll be braiding your f***ing hair with pink ribbons next, you friggin' cream-puff!

Newsflash, Kermit. There have *always* been toxins in the air; in the food we eat, the water we drink. Christ, when life first flourished, the planet was a seething volcanic chaos of poison gases like ammonia and methane. Times have been tough for life on earth since day one. That's what makes us evolve. Modern fitness writers jaw on and on about the healthy "paleo" lifestyle as if it was some kind of toxin-free paradise, but if you actually ask an archaeologist they'll tell you that this is just bullshit. Lungs of mummified bodies from the Paleolithic era are typically *black*. This is because many of our ancestors lived in caves choked with smoke and soot from constant fires, kept going for cooking, warmth, and to keep away pests and predators. Our ancient ancestors were victims to all kinds of pollution. A surprising number of early humans have been found who died from lead poisoning, for example; if there was a seam of exposed lead in the pond you drank from, that was it. You wuz pushing up flowers. And you're telling me today's environment is too "polluted" for us to match these hairy dead bastards?!

Folks also argue that our modern food is too contaminated with toxins to allow us to get the nutrition we need to make the right hormones. It's true that in the past, our forerunners had more natural food (when they could get *any* food), and they weren't force-fed synthetic high-carb foods all day. But if you reckon foods back in the day were somehow perfect, you are not in possession of the facts, my man! Much of the food consumed by bodybuilders and strongmen of the Golden Age, a hundred years and more ago, would not pass FDA approval today—in fact, it would be illegal. In Victorian England bakers added *alum*—aluminum poison—to bread, as a preservative. To hide the stench when milk went rancid, dairy farmers often poured generous amounts of *boracic acid* into their product. Highly toxic *carbolic acid* was added to almost all soap. Food was stored in lead cans, gas lighting gave off choking sulphuric vapors, and practically every building had lethal asbestos in it. Yet the men who ate this food and lived in this environment thrived and achieved things which the modern generation wouldn't even attempt without help from a pill or syringe.

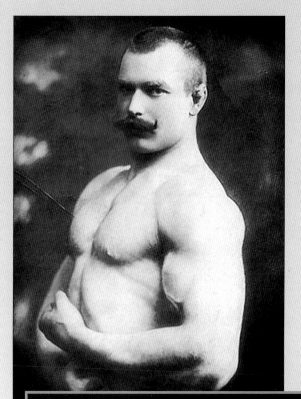

Most Victorian strongmen had enough testosterone to chew up the average modern male, and spit him in the trash. But this had nothing to do with a magically clean environment, or perfect nutrition.

It makes me laugh when modern writers go on and on about how industrial-level food production has left us with a devastating lack of nutrition in modern food. As if our ancestors somehow all had these fantasy diets. My ass! These writers don't seem to realize that before the last century—yeah, before the Industrial Revolution made food cheaper and more plentiful—one of the most common causes of death in our species was *malnutrition*! Huge swathes of the population struggled to get enough quality food in their diets to make their brains, hearts and lungs work another day, let alone grow eighteen-inch arms. It's still the same in much of the world right now. We are one of the first generations of our entire species—of any species, ever—to have such ready access to virtually limitless amounts of varied, nutrient-dense food. (That's why everyone is so friggin fat...our caveman DNA still can't quite believe we've done it.) True malnutrition in the First World is so rare today as to be virtually unheard of. So stop wringing your hands worrying if you are getting enough nutrients. Eat a steak, have a Coke and a smile, and shut the f*** up!

LIGHTS OUT!

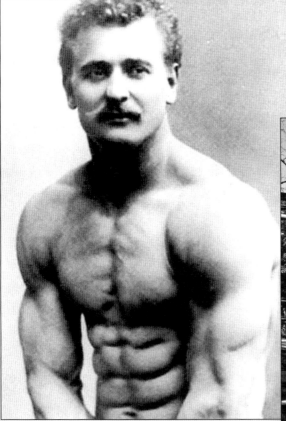

One final thought, for any bodyweight athletes who have bought into the bullshit that modern men cannot build strength or muscle without drugs. A picture is worth a thousand words, right? So let's end with a couple photos:

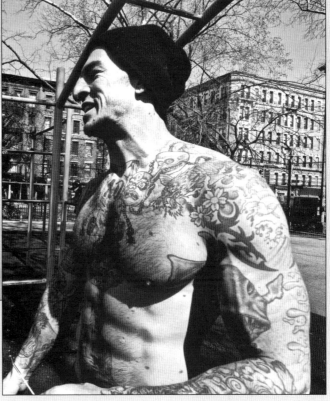

The guy top left is the infamous Eugen Sandow (b. 1867). Sandow is considered by many to be the first ever bodybuilder, and arguably owned the greatest pre-steroid physique of all time. His likeness still informs the Mr Olympia trophy. TRT/steroid fans will try and tell you that it's *impossible* to have a physique like Sandow in the modern era, due to all the toxins and pollutants that are around today.

To the right is an impromptu shot of modern bodyweight great, Danny Kavadlo, Master PCC. Danny lives and trains (usually outside) in the "polluted" air of New York City. Not only has Danny never taken *steroids*, he doesn't even take *supplements*. Danny stacks up pretty well next to Sandow, huh? In fact, I think he takes him on pecs! Does Danny look like he's low on testosterone?

If Danny can do it today…why can't *you*?

THANKS!

John Du Cane—for agreeing to promote this book and have it designed. You really are the most influential force in fitness and a true friend to me. Thank you Boss!
www.dragondoor.com

Al Kavadlo and Danny Kavadlo. These guys are becoming known all over as the best calisthenics coaches in the world. What you might not see behind their success is that these two dudes are genuinely incredible human beings who give a *huge* amount back to the bodyweight and fitness world. They donated almost all the photos in this book. Guys, you rock.
www.alkavadlo.com
www.dannythetrainer.com

Thanks to the lovely *Adrienne "Girya Girl" Harvey* for agreeing to my request and letting me publish the wonderful photo of her.
www.giryagirl.com

Max Shank is also the model in several photos here, and my thanks go out to that kid for just being generally awesome.
www.maxshank.com

Please note that all the photos donated to this project were done so *before* the text was finished…that means if you are revolted by my salty language, offensive comments, or if you plain think my ideas suck balls, the blame is mine—nobody else's!

Derek Brigham—as ever, you really are the best at what you do. If this book looks great, that's down to Big D. (Hell, if the book makes *sense*, it's down to him.)
www.dbrigham.com

And finally, thanks to all the great bodybuilders and wannabe-great bodybuilders for taking a look at C-MASS. It means a lot to me. If you want more stuff like this, head over to the *PCC blog*. Please come say hi—I hope the team will see you at a one of the bodyweight certs someday!
pccblog.dragondoor.com

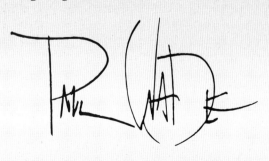

Get Harder, Stronger, More Powerful and Ripped to Shreds—with PCC, the World's Premier Bodyweight Exercise Training Program

Based on the teachings of Convict Conditioning founder, PAUL WADE… led by AL and DANNY KAVADLO

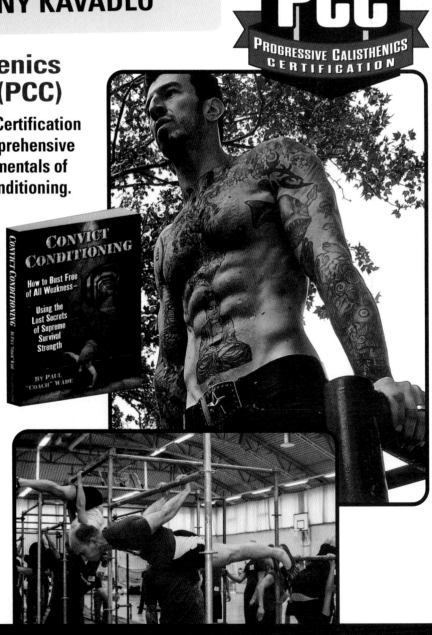

The Progressive Calisthenics Certification Workshop (PCC)

Dragon Door's Progressive Calisthenics Certification (PCC) provides you the world's most comprehensive training in the core principles and fundamentals of bodyweight exercise for strength and conditioning.

Master the cutting-edge bodyweight exercise progressions developed by *Convict Conditioning* founder **Paul Wade**—and earn the right to teach this acclaimed system to athletes, martial artists, trainers, coaches and all men and women dedicated to the cultivation of supreme strength and rugged toughness.

→ **Discover how** to generate tigrish power, enhance your coordination and balance, protect your joints, transform your physique, build steel-like tendon integrity and blowtorch fat from your body.

→ **Boost your value** as a coach or personal trainer. Not only are the movements extraordinarily cool— and adjustable to any skill level—they are also amongst the most effective, functional techniques on earth.

→ **The PCC** represents the *ultimate bodyweight cert,* and whatever your field or specialization—from strength training to rehab, bodybuilding to team sports—you will come away from this three-day cert with vast resources of training knowledge unavailable anywhere else.

The Best Training Resolution You Can Make: Log Yourself—All Year Long!

The Fastest Way to Make Physical Progress a Guarantee—Besides Dedicated, Skillful Practice—Is to Keep a Training Log

We've all heard the phrase 'the spirit is willing but the flesh is weak'. And never was this more true than in the quest for strength!

So, what are the two golden keys, or secrets to bending the flesh to the spirit's desire?

The first secret is the system—and the system is dedicated, organized application over time. And in the hard world of strength that means keeping track of your goals and measuring your progress. When it comes to serious training, you keep a log or you fail. The sins of sloppiness, haphazardness, laziness and disorganization lay waste to our dreams of physical achievement—and sabotage the best intentions to beat our flesh into righteous steel. We invite you to exorcise the demons of weakness from your flesh—with a "religious" dedication to tracking and measuring—*Convict Conditioning* style.

The second secret for strength success is inspiration. In this stunning companion to his best-selling bodyweight exercise masterpieces, Convict Conditioning author Paul Wade, goes far, far beyond the traditional log book—by delivering a bucket-load of inspiring stories and jewel-like training tips to push you forward in your quest for ever-greater strength.

This book is the first-ever training log designed specifically for bodyweight athletes. Other logs are structured to contain sections where you detail the amount of weight you used, the type of equipment or machine you worked out on, even what your heart-rate was and what vitamins you took today. You won't find any of this distracting information in this log. It's a log for pure, unadulterated, hardcore bodyweight training. We provide the inspiration and the structure—you provide the perspiration and bloody-mindedness to seize the plan and make it happen.

There is a window of opportunity awaiting you. The strength gains that have continued to elude you can finally be yours. That window of opportunity lies within these pages and within your heart. Bring it!

By far the best log book we have seen, frankly, is **Paul Wade's *Convict Conditioning Ultimate Bodyweight Training Log*. But don't think that you have to use it just for your bodyweight work. It'll serve just as well to document your progress with kettlebells, martial arts or any other practice.**

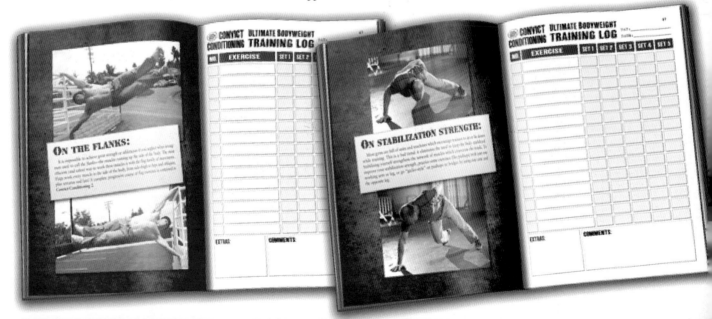

Reader Praise for *Convict Conditioning Ultimate Bodyweight Training Log*

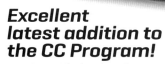

Above and Beyond!

"Not JUST a log book. TONS of great and actually useful info. I really like to over complicate programming and data entries at times. And honestly, All one has to do is fill in the blanks... Well that and DO THE WORK. Great product."
—Noel Price, Chicagoland, IL

A unique training log

"This log book is one of a kind in the world. It is the only published body weight exclusive training log I have personally seen. It is well structured and provides everything for a log book in a primarily body weight oriented routine. The book is best integrated with the other books in the convict conditioning series however has enough information to act as a stand alone unit. It is a must have for anyone who is a fan of the convict conditioning series or is entering into calisthenics." — Carter D., Cambridge, Canada

Excellent Companion to Convict Conditioning 1 & 2

"This is an amazing book! If you are a fan of Convict Conditioning (1 & 2) you need to get this training log. If you are preparing for the Progressive Calisthenics Certification then it's a must-have!!! The spiral bound format is a huge improvement over the regular binding and it makes it that much more functional for use in the gym. Great design, amazing pictures and additional content! Once again - Great job Dragon Door!"
—Michael Krivka, RKC Team Leader, Gaithersburg, MD

Excellent latest addition to the CC Program!

"A terrific book to keep you on track and beyond. Thank you again for this incredible series!"
—Joshua Hatcher, Holyoke, MA

Calling this a Log Book is Selling it Short

"I thought, what is the big deal about a logbook! Seriously mistaken. It is a work of art and with tips on each page that would be a great book all by itself. Get it. It goes way beyond a log book...the logging part of this book is just a bonus. You must have this!"—Jon Engum, Brainerd, MN

The Ultimate Bodyweight Conditioning

"I have started to incorporate bodyweight training into my strength building when I am not going to the gym. At the age of 68, after 30 years in the gym the 'Convict Conditioning Log' is going to be a welcome new training challenge."
—William Hayden, Winter Park, FL

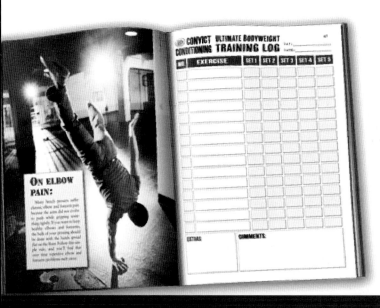

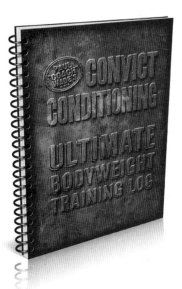

Convict Conditioning Ultimate Bodyweight Training Log

By Paul "Coach" Wade
#B67 $29.95
eBook $19.95
Paperback (spiral bound) 6 x 9
290 pages 175 photos

1 Beginner **2** Mid-Level **3** Advanced

www.dragondoor.com
1·800·899·5111
Dragon Door

Order CC Training Log online:
www.dragondoor.com/B67

How Do YOU Stack Up Against These 6 Signs of a TRUE Physical Specimen?

According to Paul Wade's *Convict Conditioning* you earn the right to call yourself a 'true physical specimen' if you can perform the following:

1. AT LEAST one set of 5 one-arm pushups each side—with the ELITE goal of 100 sets each side

2. AT LEAST one set of 5 one-leg squats each side—with the ELITE goal of 2 sets of 50 each side

3. AT LEAST a single one-arm pullup each side—with the ELITE goal of 2 sets of 6 each side

4. AT LEAST one set of 5 hanging straight leg raises—with the ELITE goal of 2 sets of 30

5. AT LEAST one stand-to-stand bridge—with the ELITE goal of 2 sets of 30

6. AT LEAST a single one-arm handstand pushup on each side— with the ELITE goal of 1 set of 5

Well, how DO you stack up?

Chances are that whatever athletic level you have achieved, there are some serious gaps in your OVERALL strength program. Gaps that stop you short of being able to claim status as a truly accomplished strength athlete.

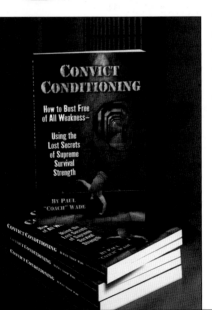

The good news is that—in *Convict Conditioning*—Paul Wade has laid out a brilliant 6-set system of 10 progressions which allows you to master these elite levels.

And you could be starting at almost any age and in almost in any condition...

Paul Wade has given you the keys—ALL the keys you'll ever need— that will open door, after door, after door for you in your quest for supreme physical excellence. Yes, it will be the hardest work you'll ever have to do. And yes, 97% of those who pick up *Convict Conditioning*, frankly, won't have the guts and the fortitude to make it. But if you make it even half-way through **Paul's Progressions**, you'll be stronger than almost anyone you encounter. Ever.

Here's just a small taste of what you'll get with *Convict Conditioning*:

Can you meet these 5 benchmarks of the *truly* powerful?... Page 1

The nature and the art of real strength... Page 2

Why mastery of *progressive calisthenics* is the ultimate secret for building maximum raw strength... Page 2

A dozen one-arm handstand pushups without support—anyone? Anyone?... Page 3

How to rank in a powerlifting championship—*without ever training with weights*... Page 4

Calisthenics as a hardcore strength training technology... Page 9

Spartan "300" calisthenics at the Battle of Thermopolylae... Page 10

How to cultivate the perfect body—the Greek and Roman way... Page 10

The difference between "old school" and "new school" calisthenics... Page 15

The role of prisons in preserving the older systems... Page 16

Strength training as a primary survival strategy... Page 16

The 6 basic benefits of bodyweight training... Pages 22—27

Why calisthenics are the *ultimate* in functional training... Page 23

The value of cultivating *self-movement*—rather than *object-movement*... Page 23

The *real* source of strength—it's not your *muscles*... Page 24

One crucial reason why a lot of convicts deliberately avoid weight-training... Page 24

How to progressively strengthen your joints over a lifetime—and even heal old joint injuries... Page 25

Why "authentic" exercises like pullups are so perfect for strength and power development... Page 25

Bodyweight training for quick physique perfection... Page 26

How to normalize and regulate your body fat levels—with body weight training only... Page 27

Why weight-training and the psychology of overeating go hand in hand... Page 27

The best approach for rapidly strengthening your whole body this... Page 30

This is the most important and revolutionary feature of *Convict Conditioning*.... Page 33

A jealously-guarded system for going from puny to powerful—when your life may depend on the speed of your results... Page 33

The 6 "Ultimate" Master Steps—only a handful of athletes in the whole world can correctly perform them all. Can you?... Page 33

How to Forge Armor-Plated Pecs and Steel Triceps... Page 41

Why the pushup is the *ultimate* upper body exercise—and better than the bench press... Page 41

How to effectively bulletproof the vulnerable rotator cuff muscles... Page 42

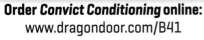

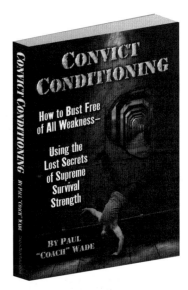

Beginner   Mid-Level   Advanced

Convict Conditioning
*How to Bust Free of
All Weakness—Using the
Lost Secrets of Supreme Survival
Strength*
By Paul "Coach" Wade
#B41 $39.95
eBook $19.95
Paperback 8.5 x 11 320 pages
191 photos, charts and illustrations

Dragon Door Customer Acclaim for Paul Wade's *Convict Conditioning*

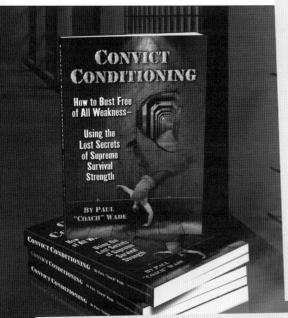

A Strength Training Guide That Will Never Be Duplicated!

"I knew within the first chapter of reading this book that I was in for something special and unique. The last time I felt this same feeling was when reading *Power to the People!* To me this is the Body Weight equivalent to Pavel's masterpiece.

Books like this can never be duplicated. Paul Wade went through a unique set of circumstances of doing time in prison with an 'old time' master of calisthenics. Paul took these lessons from this 70 year old strong man and mastered them over a period of 20 years while 'doing time'. He then taught these methods to countless prisoners and honed his teaching to perfection.

I believe that extreme circumstances like this are what it takes to create a true masterpiece. I know that 'masterpiece' is a strong word, but this is as close as it gets. No other body weight book I have read (and I have a huge fitness library)...comes close to this as far as gaining incredible strength from body weight exercise.

Just like Power to the People, I am sure I will read this over and over again...mastering the principles that Paul Wade took 20 years to master.

Outstanding Book!"—*Rusty Moore - Fitness Black Book - Seattle, WA*

A must for all martial artists

"As a dedicated martial artist for more than seven years, this book is exactly what I've been looking for.

For a while now I have trained with machines at my local gym to improve my muscle strength and power and get to the next level in my training. I always felt that the modern health club, technology based exercise jarred with my martial art though, which only required body movement.

Finally this book has come along. At last I can combine perfect body movement for martial skill with perfect body exercise for ultimate strength.

All fighting arts are based on body movement. This book is a complete textbook on how to max out your musclepower using only body movement, as different from dumbbells, machines or gadgets. For this reason it belongs on the bookshelf of every serious martial artist, male and female, young and old."—*Gino Cartier - Washington DC*

Brutal Elegance.

"I have been training and reading about training since I first joined the US Navy i the 1960s. I thought I'd seen everything the fitness world had to offer. Sometimes twice. But I was wrong. This book is utterly iconoclastic.

The author breaks down all conceivable body weight exercises into six basic mov ments, each designed to stimulate different vectors of the muscular system. These six are then elegantly and very intelligently broken into ten progressive techniques You master one technique, and move on to the next.

The simplicity of this method belies a very powerful and complex training para digm, reduced into an abstraction that obviously took many years of sweat and to to develop.

Trust me. Nobody else worked this out. This approach is completely unique and fresl

I have read virtually every calisthenics book printed in America over the last 40 years, and instruction like this can't be found anywhere, in any one of them. *Convict Conditioning* is head and shoulders above them all. In years to come, trainers and coaches will all be talking about 'progressions' and 'progressive calisthenics' and claim they've been doing it all along. But the truth is that Dragon Door bough it to you first. As with kettlebells, they were the trail blazers.

Who should purchase this volume? Everyone who craves fitness and strength should. Even if you don't plan to follow the routines, the book will make you thin! about your physical prowess, and will give even world class experts food for thought. At the very least if you find yourself on vacation or away on business without your barbells, this book will turn your hotel into a fully equipped gym.

I'd advise any athlete to obtain this work as soon as possible."—*Bill Oliver - Albany, NY, United States*

I've packed all of my other training books away!

"I read CC in one go. I couldn't put it down. I have purchased a lot of body-weight training books in the past, and have always been pretty disappointed. They all seem to just have pictures of different exercises, and no plan whatsoever on how to implement them and progress with them. But not with this one. The information in this book is AWESOME! I like to have a clear, logical plan of progression to follow, and that is what this book gives. I have put all of my other training books away. CC is the only system I am going to follow. This is now my favorite training book ever!"—*Lyndan - Australia*

More Dragon Door Customer Acclaim for *Convict Conditioning*

Fascinating Reading and Real Strength

"Coach Wade's system is a real eye opener if you've been a lifetime iron junkie. Wanna find out how really strong (or weak) you are? Get this book and begin working through the 10 levels of the 6 power exercises. I was pleasantly surprised by my ability on a few of the exercises...but some are downright humbling. If I were on a desert island with only one book on strength and conditioning this would be it. (Could I staple Pavel's "Naked Warrior" to the back and count them as one???!) Thanks Dragon Door for this innovative new author."—*Jon Schultheis, RKC (2005) - Keansburg, NJ*

Single best strength training book ever!

"I just turned 50 this year and I have tried a little bit of everything over the years: martial arts, swimming, soccer, cycling, free weights, weight machines, even yoga and Pilates. I started using *Convict Conditioning* right after it came out. I started from the beginning, like Coach Wade says, doing mostly step one or two for five out of the six exercises. I work out 3 to 5 times a week, usually for 30 to 45 minutes.

Long story short, my weight went up 14 pounds (I was not trying to gain weight) but my body fat percentage dropped two percent. That translates into approximately 19 pounds of lean muscle gained in two months! I've never gotten this kind of results with anything else I've ever done. Now I have pretty much stopped lifting weights for strength training. Instead, I lift once a week as a test to see how much stronger I'm getting without weight training. There are a lot of great strength training books in the world (most of them published by Dragon Door), but if I had to choose just one, this is the single best strength training book ever. BUY THIS BOOK. FOLLOW THE PLAN. GET AS STRONG AS YOU WANT. "—*Wayne - Decatur, GA*

Best bodyweight training book so far!

I'm a martial artist and I've been training for years with a combination of weights and bodyweight training and had good results from both (but had the usual injuries from weight training). I prefer the bodyweight stuff though as it trains me to use my whole body as a unit, much more than weights do, and I notice the difference on the mat and in the ring. Since reading this book I have given the weights a break and focused purely on the bodyweight exercise progressions as described by 'Coach' Wade and my strength had increased more than ever before. So far I've built up to 12 strict one-leg squats each leg and 5 uneven pull ups each arm.

I've never achieved this kind of strength before - and this stuff builds solid muscle mass as well. It's very intense training. I am so confident in and happy with the results I'm getting that I've decided to train for a fitness/bodybuilding comp just using his techniques, no weights, just to show for real what kind of a physique these exercises can build. In sum, I cannot recommend 'Coach' Wade's book highly enough - it is by far the best of its kind ever!"—*Mark Robinson - Australia, currently living in South Korea*

A lifetime of lifting...and continued learning.

"I have been working out diligently since 1988 and played sports in high school and college before that. My stint in the Army saw me doing calisthenics, running, conditioning courses, forced marches, etc. There are many levels of strength and fitness. I have been as big as 240 in my powerlifting/strongman days and as low as 185-190 while in the Army. I think I have tried everything under the sun: the high intensity of Arthur Jones and Dr. Ken, the Super Slow of El Darden, and the brutality of Dinosaur Training Brooks Kubic made famous.

This is one of the BEST books I've ever read on real strength training which also covers other just as important aspects of health; like staying injury free, feeling healthy and becoming flexible. It's an excellent book. He tells you the why and the how with his progressive plan. This book is a GOLD MINE and worth 100 times what I paid for it!"
—*Horst - Woburn, MA*

This book sets the standard, ladies and gentlemen

"It's difficult to describe just how much this book means to me. I've been training hard since I was in the RAF nearly ten years ago, and to say this book is a breakthrough is an understatement. How often do you really read something so new, so fresh? This book contains a complete new system of calisthenics drawn from American prison training methods. When I say 'system' I mean it. It's complete (rank beginner to expert), it's comprehensive (all the exercises and photos are here), it's graded (progressions from exercise to exercise are smooth and pre-determined) and it's totally original. Whether you love or hate the author, you have to listen to him. And you will learn something. This book just makes SENSE. In twenty years people will still be buying it."—*Andy McMann - Ponty, Wales, GB*

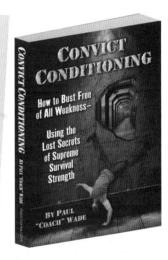

Convict Conditioning
How to Bust Free of All Weakness—Using the Lost Secrets of Supreme Survival Strength
By Paul "Coach" Wade
#B41 $39.95
eBook $19.95
Paperback 8.5 x 11 320 pages
191 photos, charts and illustrations

1 Beginner **2** Mid-Level **3** Advanced

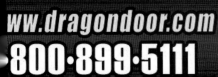

The Experts Give High Praise to
Convict Conditioning 2

"Coach Paul Wade has outdone himself. His first book *Convict Conditioning* is to my mind THE BEST book ever written on bodyweight conditioning. Hands down. Now, with the sequel *Convict Conditioning 2*, Coach Wade takes us even deeper into the subtle nuances of training with the ultimate resistance tool: our bodies.

In plain English, but with an amazing understanding of anatomy, physiology, kinesiology and, go figure, psychology, Coach Wade explains very simply how to work the smaller but just as important areas of the body such as the hands and forearms, neck and calves and obliques in serious functional ways.

His minimalist approach to exercise belies the complexity of his system and the deep insight into exactly how the body works and the best way to get from A to Z in the shortest time possible.

I got the best advice on how to strengthen the hard-to-reach extensors of the hand right away from this exercise Master I have ever seen. It's so simple but so completely functional I can't believe no one else has thought of it yet. Just glad he figured it out for me.

Paul teaches us how to strengthen our bodies with the simplest of movements while at the same time balancing our structures in the same way: simple exercises that work the whole body.

And just as simply as he did with his first book. His novel approach to stretching and mobility training is brilliant and fresh as well as his take on recovery and healing from injury. Sprinkled throughout the entire book are too-many-to-count insights and advice from a man who has come to his knowledge the hard way and knows exactly of what he speaks.

This book is, as was his first, an amazing journey into the history of physical culture disguised as a book on calisthenics. But the thing that Coach Wade does better than any before him is his unbelievable progressions on EVERY EXERCISE and stretch! He breaks things down and tells us EXACTLY how to proceed to get to whatever level of strength and development we want. AND gives us the exact metrics we need to know when to go to the next level.

Adding in completely practical and immediately useful insights into nutrition and the mindset necessary to deal not only with training but with life, makes this book a classic that will stand the test of time.

Bravo Coach Wade, Bravo." —**Mark Reifkind**, Master RKC, author of *Mastering the HardStyle Kettlebell Swing*

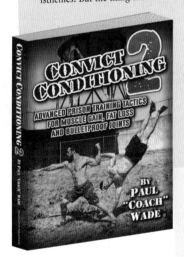

Convict Conditioning 2
Advanced Prison Training Tactics for Muscle Gain, Fat Loss and Bulletproof Joints
By Paul "Coach" Wade
#B59 $39.95
eBook $19.95
Paperback 8.5 x 11 354 pages
261 photos, charts and illustrations

2 Mid-Level

3 Advanced

"The overriding principle of *Convict Conditioning 2* is 'little equipment-big rewards'. For the athlete in the throwing and fighting arts, the section on Lateral Chain Training, Capturing the Flag, is a unique and perhaps singular approach to training the obliques and the whole family of side muscles. This section stood out to me as ground breaking and well worth the time and energy by anyone to review and attempt to complete. Literally, this is a new approach to lateral chain training that is well beyond sidebends and suitcase deadlifts.

The author's review of passive stretching reflects the experience of many of us in the field. But, his solution might be the reason I am going to recommend this work for everyone: The Trifecta. This section covers what the author calls The Functional Triad and gives a series of simple progressions to three holds that promise to oil your joints. It's yoga for the strength athlete and supports the material one would find, for example, in Pavel's *Loaded Stretching*.

I didn't expect to like this book, but I come away from it practically insisting that everyone read it. It is a strongman book mixed with yoga mixed with street smarts. I wanted to hate it, but I love it."
—**Dan John**, author of *Don't Let Go* and co-author of *Easy Strength*

"I've been lifting weights for over 50 years and have trained in the martial arts since 1965. I've read voraciously on both subjects, and written dozens of magazine articles and many books on the subjects. This book and Wade's first, *Convict Conditioning*, are by far the most commonsense, information-packed, and result producing I've read. These books will truly change your life.

Paul Wade is a new and powerful voice in the strength and fitness arena, one that is commonsense, inspiring, and in your face. His approach to maximizing your body's potential is not the same old hackneyed material you find in every book and magazine piece that pictures steroid-bloated models screaming as they curl weights. Wade's stuff has been proven effective by hard men who don't tolerate fluff. It will work for you, too—guaranteed.

As an ex-cop, I've gone mano-y-mano with ex-cons that had clearly trained as Paul Wade suggests in his two *Convict Conditioning* books. While these guys didn't look like steroid-fueled bodybuilders (actually, there were a couple who did), all were incredibly lean, hard and powerful. Wade blows many commonly held beliefs about conditioning, strengthening, and eating out of the water and replaces them with result-producing information that won't cost you a dime." —**Loren W. Christensen**, author of *Fighting the Pain Resistant Attacker,* and many other titles

"*Convict Conditioning* is one of the most influential books I ever got my hands on. *Convict Conditioning 2* took my training and outlook on the power of bodyweight training to the 10th degree—from strengthening the smallest muscles in a maximal manner, all the way to using bodyweight training as a means of healing injuries that pile up from over 22 years of aggressive lifting.

I've used both *Convict Conditioning* and *Convict Conditioning 2* on myself and with my athletes. Without either of these books I can easily say that these boys would not be the BEASTS they are today. Without a doubt *Convict Conditioning 2* will blow you away and inspire and educate you to take bodyweight training to a whole NEW level."
—**Zach Even-Esh**, Underground Strength Coach

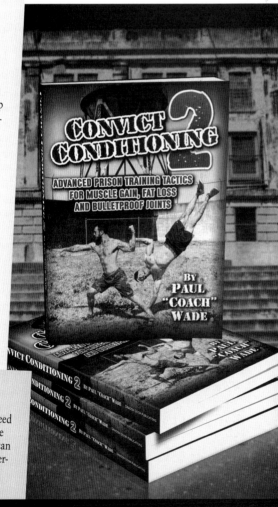

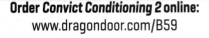

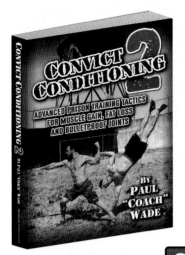

Convict Conditioning 2

Advanced Prison Training Tactics for Muscle Gain, Fat Loss and Bulletproof Joints

By Paul "Coach" Wade
#B59 $39.95
eBook $19.95

Paperback 8.5 x 11 354 pages
261 photos, charts and illustrations

2 Mid-Level

3 Advanced

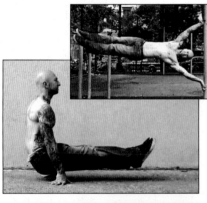

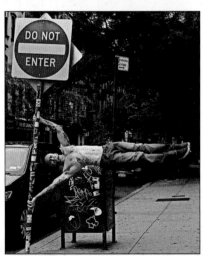

TABLE OF CONTENTS

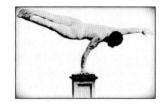
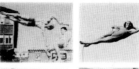

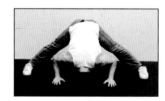
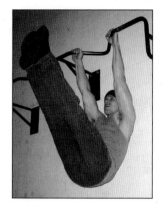
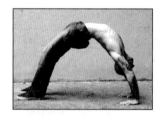
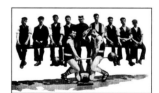

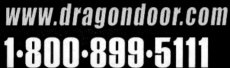

GET DYNAMIC, CHISELLED, POWER-JACK LEGS AND DEVELOP EXPLOSIVE LOWER-BODY STRENGTH— WITH PAUL "COACH" WADE'S ULTIMATE BODYWEIGHT SQUAT COURSE

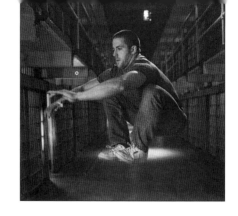

Paul Wade's *Convict Conditioning Ultimate Bodyweight Squat Course* explodes out of the cellblock to teach you in absolute detail how to progress from the ease of a simple shoulderstand squat—to the stunning "1-in-10,000" achievement of the prison-style one-leg squat. Ten progressive steps guide you to bodyweight squat mastery. Do it—and become a Bodyweight Squat Immortal.

This home-study course in ultimate survival strength comes replete with bonus material not available in **Paul Wade's** original *Convict Conditioning* book—and numerous key training tips that refine and expand on the original program.

A heavily and gorgeously-illustrated 80-plus-page manual gives you the entire film script to study at your leisure, with brilliant, precise photographs to remind you of the essential movements you absorbed in the DVD itself.

Paul Wade adds a bonus **Ten Commandments for Perfect Bodyweight Squats**—which is worth the price of admission alone. And there's the additional bonus of **5 major Variant drills** to add explosivity, fun and super-strength to your core practice.

Whatever you are looking for from your bodyweight squats—be it supreme functional strength, monstrous muscle growth or explosive leg power—it's yours for the progressive taking with *Convict Conditioning, Volume 2: The Ultimate Bodyweight Squat Course.*

WHY EVERY SELF-RESPECTING MAN WILL BE RELIGIOUS ABOUT HIS SQUATS...

Leg training is vital for every athlete. A well-trained, muscular upper body teetering around on skinny stick legs is a joke. Don't be that joke! The mighty squat is the answer to your prayers. Here's why:

- Squats train virtually every muscle in the lower body, from quads and glutes to hips, lower back and even hamstrings.

- Squat deep—as we'll teach you—and you will seriously increase your flexibility and ankle strength.

- All functional power is transmitted through the legs, so without strong, powerful legs you are *nothing*—that goes for running, jumping and combat sports as much as it does for lifting heavy stuff.

ARE YOU FAILING TO BUILD MONSTROUS LEGS FROM SQUATS—BECAUSE OF THESE MISTAKES?

Most trainees learn how to squat on two legs, and then make the exercise harder by slapping a barbell across their back. In prison, this way of adding strength wasn't always available, so cell trainees developed ways of progressing using only bodyweight versus gravity. The best way to do this is to learn how to squat all the way down to the ground and back up on just one leg.

Not everybody who explores prison training will have the dedication and drive to achieve strength feats like the one-arm pullup, but the legs are much stronger than the arms. If you put in the time and work hard, the one-leg squat will be within the reach of almost every athlete who pays their dues.

But the one-leg squat still requires very powerful muscles and tendons, so you don't want to jump into one-leg squatting right away. You need to build the joint strength and muscle to safely attempt this great exercise. Discover how to do that safely, using ten steps, ten progressively harder squat exercises.

IN THE STRENGTH GAME, FOOLS RUSH IN WHERE ANGELS FEAR TO TREAD

The wise old Chinese man shouted to his rickshaw driver: "Slow down, young man, I'm in a hurry!" If ever a warning needed to be shouted to our nation of compulsive strength-addicts, this would be it. You see them everywhere: the halt, the lame, the jacked-up, the torn, the pain-ridden—the former glory-seekers who have been reduced to sad husks of their former selves by rushing helter-skelter into heavy lifting without having first built a firm foundation.

Paul Wade reveals the ten key points of perfect squat form. The aspects of proper form apply to all your squats, and they'll not only unlock the muscle and power-building potential of each rep you do, but they'll also keep you as safe as you can be.

Bodyweight training is all about improving strength and health, not building up a list of injuries or aches and pains. They are so fundamental, we call them the Ten Commandments of good squat form.

Obey the Ten Commandments, follow the brilliantly laid out progressions religiously and you simply CANNOT fail to get stronger and stronger and stronger and stronger and stronger—surely, safely and for as long as you live…

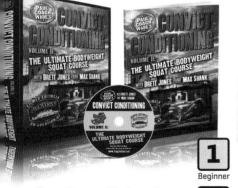

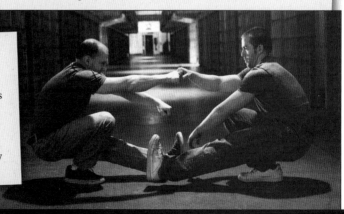

GET A ROCK-HARD, BRUTISHLY POWERFUL UPPER FRAME AND ACHIEVE ELITE-LEVEL STRENGTH—WITH PAUL "COACH" WADE'S PRISON-STYLE PUSHUP PROGRAM

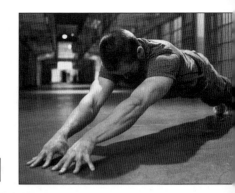

Paul Wade's *Convict Conditioning* system represents the ultimate distillation of hardcore prison bodyweight training's most powerful methods. What works was kept. What didn't, was slashed away. When your life is on the line, you're not going to mess with less than the absolute best. Many of these older, very potent solitary training systems have been on the verge of dying, as convicts begin to gain access to weights, and modern "bodybuilding thinking" floods into the prisons.

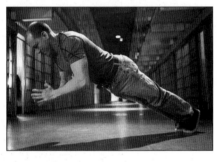

Thanks to Paul Wade, these ultimate strength survival secrets have been saved for posterity. And for you...

Filmed entirely—and so appropriately—on "The Rock", Wade's *Convict Conditioning Prison Pushup Series* explodes out of the cellblock to teach you in absolute detail how to progress from the ease of a simple wall pushup—to the stunning "1-in-10,000" achieve-ment of the prison-style one-arm pushup. Ten progressive steps guide you to pushup mastery. Do it—and become a Pushup God.

This home-study course in ultimate survival strength comes replete with bonus material not available in **Paul Wade's** original *Convict Conditioning* book—and numerous key training tips that refine and expand on the original program.

A heavily and gorgeously-illustrated 80-plus-page manual gives you the entire film script to study at your leisure, with brilliant, precise photographs to remind you of the essential movements you absorbed in the DVD itself.

Paul Wade adds a bonus **Ten Commandments for Perfect Pushups**—which is worth the price of admission alone. And there's the additional bonus of **5 major Variant drills** to add explosivity, fun and super-strength to your core practice.

Whatever you are looking for from your pushups—be it supreme functional strength, monstrous muscle growth or explosive upper-body power—it's yours for the progressive taking with *Convict Conditioning, Volume 1: The Prison Pushup Series.*

AWESOME RESOURCE FOR COACHES & STRENGTH DEVOTEES

"I am using this manual and DVD not just for my own training, but for the training of my athletes. It shocks and amazes me how varsity high school athletes can NOT perform a solid push up.... not even 1! Getting them to perform a perfect push up requires regressions, progressions, dialing in the little cues that teach them to generate tension and proper body alignment, ALL of which carry over to other exercises.

This manual is an awesome resource for Coaches. It can & should be used to educate those you train as well as shared with your staff. For those who have a love for strength, you will respect all the details given for each and every push up pro-gression and you will use them and apply them.

As a Strength devotee for over 2 decades, I've been through the grinder with free weights and injuries, push ups are something I KNOW I'll be doing for the rest of my life which is why I RESPECT this course so much!

The lay out of this manual and DVD are also BIG time impressive, the old school look and feel fires me up and makes me wanna attack these push ups!"
—Zach Even-Esh, Manasquan, NJ

I RECOMMEND IT

"I fully expected to be disappointed with **Paul Wade's** *Convict Conditioning, Volume 1: The Prison Pushup Series*. John Du Cane will tell you: I am not a fan of some of the stuff in these books. It's been said by others that this might be one of the most striking DVDs ever made. It's on location in Alcatraz and the graphic are pretty amazing. So, yes, stunning. This DVD from Wade is stunning and very cool.

The manual that supports the DVD is very helpful as much of the material is done too well in the DVD. Many of us need to take some time looking at the DVD then flipping the manual back and forth to 'get it.'

Once again, there are parts of this DVD and the series that rub me the wrong way. Having said that, I am frankly amazed at the insights of the product here. As a coach, I am better than when I popped the box open. I have a whole set of tools, and the progressions, that I can use tomorrow with my group. That to me the testimony that people should hear from me: I watched it and I applied it instantly! This one 'gets it.' You can apply what you learn instantly know where you are going from there. I highly recommend it."
—Dan John, Master RKC, Burlingame, CA

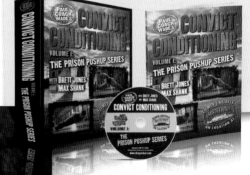

Convict Conditioning
Volume 1: The Prison Pushup Series
By Paul "Coach" Wade featuring Brett Jones and Max Shank
#DV083 $69.95
DVD 59 minutes with full color Companion Manual, 88 pages

1 Beginner

2 Mid-Level

3 Advanced

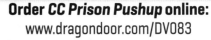

DEMONIC ABS ARE A MAN'S BEST FRIEND—DISCOVER HOW TO SEIZE A SIX-PACK FROM HELL AND OWN THE WORLD...
LEG RAISES

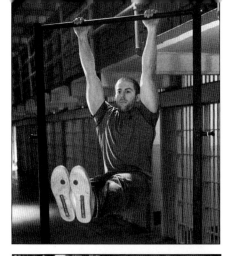

Paul Wade's *Convict Conditioning 3, Leg Raises: Six Pack from Hell* teaches you in absolute detail how to progress from the ease of a simple Knee Tuck—to the magnificent, "1-in-1,000" achievement of the Hanging Straight Leg Raise. Ten progressive steps guide you to inevitable mastery of this ultimate abs exercise. Do it, seize the knowledge—but beware—the Gods will be jealous!

This home-study course in ultimate survival strength comes replete with bonus material not available in **Paul** Wade's original *Convict Conditioning* book—and numerous key training tips that refine and expand on the original program.

Prowl through the heavily and gorgeously-illustrated 80-plus-page manual and devour the entire film script at your animal leisure. Digest the brilliant, precise photographs and reinforce the raw benefits you absorbed from the DVD.

Paul Wade adds a bonus **Ten Commandments for Perfect Bodyweight Squats**—which is worth the price of admission alone. And there's the additional bonus of **4 major Variant drills** to add explosivity, fun and super-strength to your core practice.

Whatever you are looking for when murdering your abs—be it a fist-breaking, rock-like shield of impenetrable muscle, an uglier-is-more-beautiful set of rippling abdominal ridges, or a monstrous injection of lifting power—it's yours for the progressive taking with *Convict Conditioning, Volume 3, Leg Raises: Six Pack from Hell*

PRISON-STYLE MID-SECTION TRAINING— FOR AN ALL SHOW AND ALL GO PHYSIQUE

When convicts train their waists, they want real, noticeable results—and by "results" we don't mean that they want cute, tight little defined abs. We mean that they want thick, strong, muscular midsections. They want *functionally* powerful abs and hips they can use for heavy lifting, kicking, and brawling. They want guts so strong from their training that it actually hurts an attacker to punch them in the belly. Prison abs aren't about all show, no go—a prison-built physique has to be all show and all go. Those guys don't just want six-packs—they want six-packs from Hell.

And, for the first time, we're going to show you how these guys get what they want. We're not going to be using sissy machines or easy isolation exercises—we're going straight for the old school secret weapon for gut training; progressive leg raises.

If you want a six-pack from Hell, the first thing you need to do is focus your efforts. If a weightlifter wanted a very thick, powerful chest in a hurry, he wouldn't spread his efforts out over a dozen exercises and perform them gently all day long. No—he'd pick just one exercise, probably the bench press, and just focus on getting stronger and stronger on that lift until he was monstrously strong. When he reached this level, and his pecs were thick slabs of meat, only then would he maybe begin sculpting them with minor exercises and higher reps.

It's no different if you want a mind-blowing midsection. Just pick one exercise that hits all the muscles in the midsection—the hip flexors, the abs, the intercostals, the obliques—then blast it.

And the one exercise we're going to discover is the best midsection exercise known to man, and the most popular amongst soldiers, warriors, martial artists and prison athletes since men started working out—the leg raise.

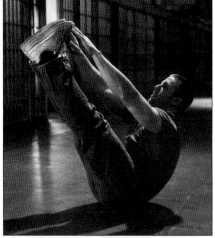

You'll discover ten different leg raise movements, each one a little harder than the last. You'll learn how to get the most out of each of these techniques, each of these ten steps, before moving up to the next step. By the time you get through all ten steps and you're working with the final Master Step of the leg raise series, you'll have a solid, athletic, stomach made of steel, as well as powerful hips and a ribcage armored with dense muscle. You'll have abs that would've made Bruce Lee take notice!

THE TEN COMMANDMENTS YOU MUST OBEY TO EARN A REAL MONSTER OF AN ATHLETIC CORE

Paul Wade gives you ten key points, the "Ten Commandments" of leg raises, that will take your prison-style core training from just "okay" to absolutely phenomenal. We want the results to be so effective that they'll literally shock you. This kind of accelerated progress can be achieved, but if you want to achieve it you better listen carefully to these ten key pointers you'll discover with the DVD.

Bodyweight mastery is a lot like high-level martial arts. It's more about *principles* than individual techniques. Really study and absorb these principles, and you'll be on your way to a six-pack from Hell in no time.

The hanging straight leg raise, performed strictly and for reps, is the Gold Standard of abdominal strength techniques. Once you're at the level where you can throw out sets of twenty to thirty rock solid reps of this exercise, your abs will be thick and strong, but more importantly, they'll be functional—not just a pretty six-pack, but a real monster of an athletic core, which is

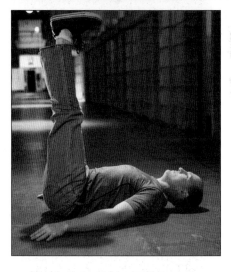

capable of developing high levels of force.

Hanging will work your serratus and intercostals, making these muscles stand out like fingers, and your obliques and flank muscles will be tight and strong from holding your hips in place. Your lumbar spine will achieve a gymnastic level of flexibility, like fluid steel, and your chances of back pain will be greatly reduced.

The bottom line: If you want to be stronger and more athletic than the next guy, you need the edge that straight leg raises can give you.

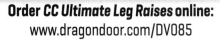

ERECT TWIN PYTHONS OF COILED BEEF UP YOUR SPINE AND DEVELOP EXTREME, EXPLOSIVE RESILIENCE—WITH THE DYNAMIC POWER AND FLEXIBLE STRENGTH OF
ADVANCED BRIDGING

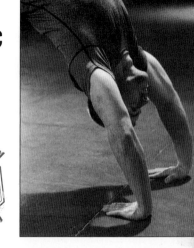

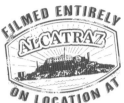

P aul Wade's *Convict Conditioning* system represents the ultimate distillation of hardcore prison bodyweight training's most powerful methods. What works was kept. What didn't, was slashed away. When your life is on the line, you're not going to mess with less than the absolute best. Many of these older, very potent solitary training systems have been on the verge of dying, as convicts begin to gain access to weights, and modern "bodybuilding thinking" floods into the prisons. Thanks to Paul Wade, these ultimate strength survival secrets have been saved for posterity. And for you...

Filmed entirely—and so appropriately— on "The Rock", Wade's *Convict Conditioning Volume 4, Advanced Bridging: Forging an Iron Spine* explodes out of the cellblock to teach you in absolute detail how to progress from the relative ease of a Short Bridge—to the stunning, "1-in-1,000" achievement of the Stand-to-Stand Bridge. Ten progressive steps guide you to inevitable mastery of this ultimate exercise for an unbreakable back.

This home-study course in ultimate sur-

vival strength comes replete with bonus material not available in **Paul Wade's** original *Convict Conditioning* book—and numerous key training tips that refine and expand on the original program.

Prowl through the heavily and gorgeously-illustrated 80-plus-page manual and devour the entire film script at your animal leisure. Digest the brilliant, precise photographs and reinforce the raw benefits you absorbed from the DVD.

Paul Wade adds a bonus **Ten Commandments for Perfect Bridges**— which is worth the price of admission alone. And there's the additional bonus of **4 major Variant drills** to add explosivity, fun and super-strength to your core practice.

Whatever you are looking for from your pushups—be it supreme functional strength, monstrous muscle growth or explosive upper-body power—it's yours for the progressive taking with *Convict Conditioning Volume 4: Advanced Bridging: Forging an Iron Spine.*

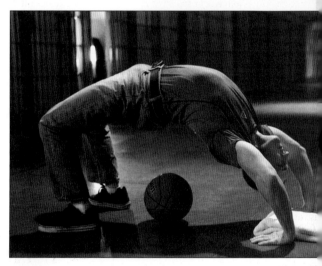

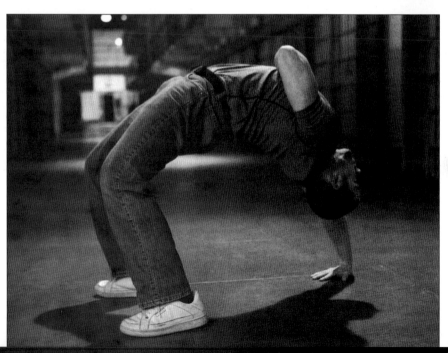

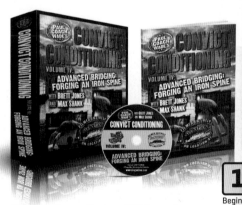

Convict Conditioning
Volume 4: Advanced Bridging: Forging an Iron Spine
By Paul "Coach" Wade featuring Brett Jones and Max Shank
#DV087 $59.95
DVD 59 minutes with full color Companion Manual, 88 pages

1 Begin

2 Mid-L

3 Advan

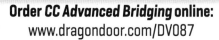

TAP INTO THE DORMANT ANCESTRAL POWER OF THE MIGHTY PULLUP—
TO DEVELOP A MASSIVE UPPER BACK, STEEL-TENDON ARMS, ETCHED ABS AND AGILE SURVIVAL STRENGTH

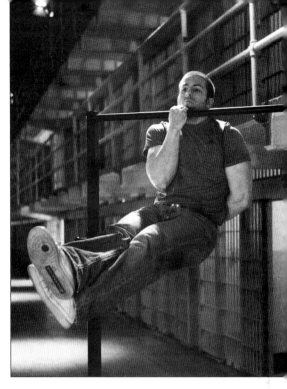

Paul Wade's *Convict Conditioning* system represents the ultimate distillation of hardcore prison bodyweight training's most powerful methods. What works was kept. What didn't, was slashed away. When your life is on the line, you're not going to mess with less than the absolute best. Many of these older, very potent solitary training systems have been on the verge of dying, as convicts begin to gain access to weights, and modern "bodybuilding thinking" floods into the prisons. Thanks to Paul Wade, these ultimate strength survival secrets have been saved for posterity. And for you…

Filmed entirely—and so appropriately— on "The Rock", Wade's *Convict Conditioning Volume 5, Maximum Strength: The One-Arm Pullup Series* explodes out of the cellblock to teach you in absolute detail how to progress from the relative ease of a Vertical Pull—to the stunning, "1-in-1,000" achievement of the One-Arm Pullup. Ten progressive steps guide you to inevitable mastery of this ultimate exercise for supreme upper body survival strength.

This home-study course in ultimate survival strength comes replete with bonus material not available in **Paul Wade's** original *Convict Conditioning* book—and numerous key training tips that refine and expand on the original program.

Prowl through the heavily and gorgeously-illustrated 80-plus-page manual and devour the entire film script at your animal leisure. Digest the brilliant, precise photographs and reinforce the raw benefits you absorbed from the DVD.

Paul Wade adds a bonus **Ten Commandments for Perfect Pullups**—which is worth the price of admission alone. And there's the additional bonus of **4 major Variant drills** to add explosivity, fun and super-strength to your core practice.

Whatever you are looking for from your pullups—be it agile survival strength, arms of steel, a massive upper back with flaring lats, Popeye Biceps or gape-inducing abs—it's yours for the progressive taking with *Convict Conditioning Volume 5, Maximum Strength: The One-Arm Pullup Series.*

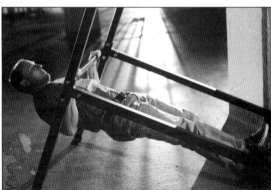

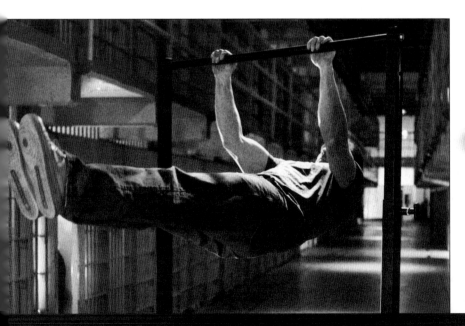

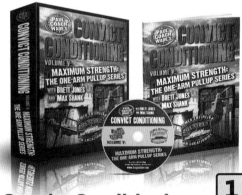

Al Kavadlo's Progressive Plan for Primal Body Power

How to Build Explosive Strength and a Magnificent Physique—Using Bodyweight Exercise Only

What is more satisfying than owning a primally powerful, functionally forceful and brute-strong body? A body that packs a punch. A body that commands attention with its etched physique, coiled muscle and proud confidence…A body that can PERFORM at the highest levels of physical accomplishment…

Well, both **Al Kavadlo**—the author of *Pushing the Limits!*—and his brother **Danny**, are supreme testaments to the primal power of body culture done the old-school, ancient way—bare-handed, with your body only. The brothers Kavadlo walk the bodyweight talk—and then

some. The proof is evident on every page of *Pushing the Limits!*

Your body is your temple. Protect and strengthen your temple by modeling the methods of the exercise masters. Al Kavadlo has modeled the masters and has the "temple" to show for it. Follow Al's progressive plan for primal body power within the pages of *Pushing the Limits!*—follow in the footsteps of the great bodyweight exercise masters—and you too can build the explosive strength and possess the magnificent physique you deserve.

> "When people ask me about bodyweight strength training, I point them to Al Kavadlo. Pushing the Limits! is a must-have for bodyweight training enthusiasts or anyone looking to build strength without lifting weights. Al lays out dozens of effective exercises for every fitness level, while making the journey fun and encouraging."
> **—MARK SISSON**, author of *The Primal Blueprint*

> "In this awesome new book, Al only asks that you find ONE piece of equipment—your body! Stoic, Spartan, perfection…this book is bodyweight strength training for the ultimate purist!"—**PAUL WADE**, author of *Convict Conditioning*

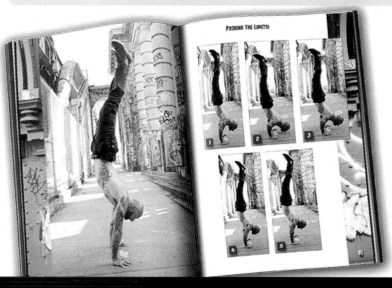

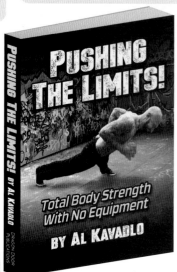

Pushing the Limits!
Total Body Strength With No Equipment
By Al Kavadlo
#B69 $39.95
eBook $19.95
Paperback 8.5 x 11 224 pages
240 photos

 1 Beginner **2** Mid-Level **3** Advanced

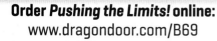

Stretching and Flexibility Secrets To Help Unlock Your Body—Be More Mobile, More Athletic, More Resilient And Far Stronger...

"The ultimate bodyweight mobility manual is here! Al Kavadlo's previous two Dragon Door books, *Raising the Bar* and *Pushing the Limits*, are the most valuable bodyweight strength training manuals in the world. But strength without mobility is meaningless. Al has used his many years of training and coaching to fuse bodyweight disciplines such as yoga, martial arts, rehabilitative therapy and bar athletics into the ultimate calisthenics stretching compendium. *Stretching your Boundaries* belongs on the shelf of any serious athlete—it's bodyweight mobility dynamite!"
— "COACH" PAUL WADE, author of *Convict Conditioning*

"In this book, Al invites you to take a deeper look at the often overlooked, and sometimes demonized, ancient practice of static stretching. He wrestles with many of the questions, dogmas and flat out lies about stretching that have plagued the fitness practitioner for at least the last decade. And finally he gives you a practical guide to static stretching that will improve your movement, performance, breathing and life. In *Stretching Your Boundaries*, you'll sense Al's deep understanding and love for the human body. Thank you Al, for helping to bring awareness to perhaps the most important aspect of physical education and fitness."
— ELLIOTT HULSE, creator of the **Grow Stronger** method

"An absolutely masterful follow up to *Raising The Bar* and *Pushing The Limits*, *Stretching Your Boundaries* really completes the picture. Both easy to understand and fully applicable, Al's integration of traditional flexibility techniques with his own unique spin makes this a must have. The explanation of how each stretch will benefit your calisthenics practice is brilliant. Not only stunning in its color and design, this book also gives you the true feeling of New York City, both gritty and euphoric, much like Al's personality."
— MIKE FITCH, creator of **Global Bodyweight Training**

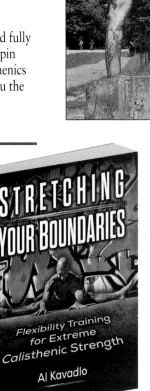

"Stretching Your Boundaries is a terrific resource that will unlock your joints so you can build more muscle, strength and athleticism. Al's passion for human performance radiates in this beautifully constructed book. Whether you're stiff as a board, or an elite gymnast, this book outlines the progressions to take your body and performance to a new level."
— CHAD WATERBURY, M.S., author of *Huge in a Hurry*

"Al Kavadlo has done it again! He's created yet another incredible resource that I wish I had twenty years ago. Finding great material on flexibility training that actually enhances your strength is like trying to find a needle in a haystack. But look no further, because *Stretching Your Boundaries* is exactly what you need."
— JASON FERRUGGIA, Strength Coach

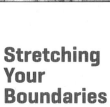

Stretching Your Boundaries
Flexibility Training for Extreme Calisthenic Strength
By Al Kavadlo
#B73 $39.95
eBook $19.95
Paperback 8.5 x 11   214 pages
235 photos

Beginner   Mid-Level   Advanced

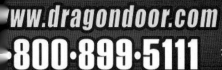

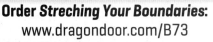

Go Beyond Mere "Toughness"— When You Master The Art of Bar Athletics and Sculpt the Ultimate in Upper Body Physiques

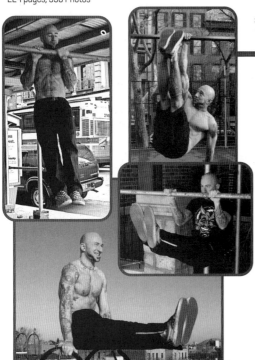
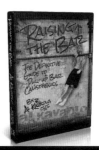

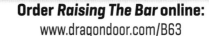

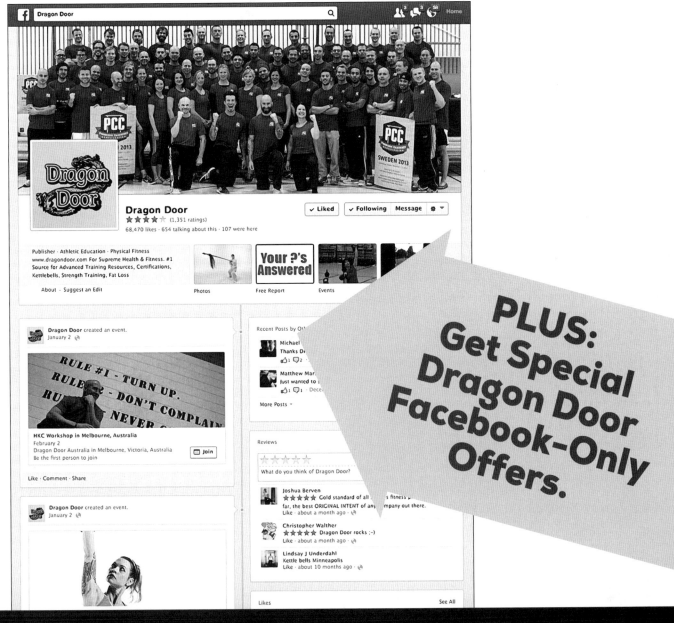

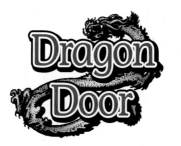

1·800·899·5111

24 HOURS A DAY • FAX YOUR ORDER (866) 280-7619

ORDERING INFORMATION

Telephone Orders For faster service you may place your orders by calling Toll Free 24 hours a day, 7 days a week, 365 days per year. When you call, please have your credit card ready.

Customer Service Questions? Please call us between 9:00am– 11:00pm EST

Monday to Friday at 1-800-899-5111. Local and foreign customers call 513-346-4160 for orders and customer service

100% One-Year Risk-Free Guarantee. If you are not completely satisfied with any product—we'll be happy to give you a prompt exchange, credit, or refund, as

you wish. Simply return your purchase to us, and please let us know why you were dissatisfied—it will help us to provide better products and services in the future. *Shipping and handling fees are non-re-fundable.*

VISA · MasterCard · AMERICAN EXPRESS Cards · DISCOVER N✩VUS

Complete and mail with full payment to: Dragon Door Publications, 5 County Road B East, Suite 3, Little Canada, MN 55117

Please print clearly

Sold To: A

Name_____

Street_____

City_____

State_____ Zip _____

Day phone*_____
* Important for clarifying questions on orders

Please print clearly

SHIP TO: *(Street address for delivery)*   B

Name_____

Street_____

City_____

State_____ Zip _____

Email_____

Warning to foreign customers

The Customs in your country may or may not tax or otherwise charge you an additional fee for goods you receive. Dragon Door Publications is charging you only for U.S. handling and international shipping. Dragon Door Publications is in no way responsible for any additional fees levied by Customs, the carrier or any other entity.

ITEM #	QTY.	ITEM DESCRIPTION	ITEM PRICE	A OR B	TOTAL

HANDLING AND SHIPPING CHARGES • NO COD'S

Total Amount of Order Add (Excludes kettlebells and kettlebell kits):

$00.00 to 29.99	Add $6.00	$100.00 to 129.99	Add $14.00
$30.00 to 49.99	Add $7.00	$130.00 to 169.99	Add $16.00
$50.00 to 69.99	Add $8.00	$170.00 to 199.99	Add $18.00
$70.00 to 99.99	Add $11.00	$200.00 to 299.99	Add $20.00
		$300.00 and up	Add $24.00

Canada and Mexico add $6.00 to US charges. All other countries, flat rate, double US Charges. See Kettlebell section for Kettlebell Shipping and handling charges.

Total of Goods	
Shipping Charges	
Rush Charges	
Kettlebell Shipping Charges	
OH residents add 6.5% sales tax	
MN residents add 6.5% sales tax	
TOTAL ENCLOSED	

METHOD OF PAYMENT ❏ CHECK ❏ M.O. ❏ MASTERCARD ❏ VISA ❏ DISCOVER ❏ AMEX

Account No. *(Please indicate all the numbers on your credit card)*   EXPIRATION DATE

☐☐☐☐ ☐☐☐☐ ☐☐☐☐ ☐☐☐☐   ☐☐/☐☐

Day Phone: (_____)_____

Signature: _____   **Date:** _____

NOTE: *We ship best method available for your delivery address. Foreign orders are sent by air. Credit card or International M.O. only. For* **RUSH** *processing of your order, add an additional $10.00 per address. Available on money order & charge card orders only.*

Errors and omissions excepted. Prices subject to change without notice.

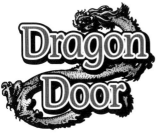

1·800·899·5111

24 HOURS A DAY • FAX YOUR ORDER (866) 280-7619

O R D E R I N G   I N F O R M A T I O N

Telephone Orders For faster service you may place your orders by calling Toll Free 24 hours a day, 7 days a week, 365 days per year. When you call, please have your credit card ready.

Customer Service Questions? Please call us between 9:00am– 11:00pm EST

Monday to Friday at 1-800-899-5111. Local and foreign customers call 513-346-4160 for orders and customer service

100% One-Year Risk-Free Guarantee. If you are not completely satisfied with any product—we'll be happy to give you a prompt exchange, credit, or refund, as

you wish. Simply return your purchase to us, and please let us know why you were dissatisfied—it will help us to provide better products and services in the future. *Shipping and handling fees are non-refundable.*

VISA MasterCard AMERICAN EXPRESS Cards DISCOVER NOVUS

Complete and mail with full payment to: Dragon Door Publications, 5 County Road B East, Suite 3, Little Canada, MN 55117

Please print clearly

Sold To: **A**

Name_____

Street_____

City_____

State_____ Zip_____

Day phone*_____
Important for clarifying questions on orders

Please print clearly

SHIP TO: *(Street address for delivery)*   **B**

Name_____

Street_____

City_____

State_____ Zip_____

Email_____

Warning to foreign customers:
The Customs in your country may or may not tax or otherwise charge you an additional fee for goods you receive. Dragon Door Publications is charging you only for U.S. handling and international shipping. Dragon Door Publications is in no way responsible for any additional fees levied by Customs, the carrier or any other entity.

ITEM #	QTY.	ITEM DESCRIPTION	ITEM PRICE	A OR B	TOTAL

HANDLING AND SHIPPING CHARGES • NO COD'S
Total Amount of Order Add (Excludes kettlebells and kettlebell kits):

$00.00 to 29.99	Add $6.00	$100.00 to 129.99	Add $14.00
$30.00 to 49.99	Add $7.00	$130.00 to 169.99	Add $16.00
$50.00 to 69.99	Add $8.00	$170.00 to 199.99	Add $18.00
$70.00 to 99.99	Add $11.00	$200.00 to 299.99	Add $20.00
		$300.00 and up	Add $24.00

Canada and Mexico add $6.00 to US charges. All other countries, flat rate, double US Charges. See Kettlebell section for Kettlebell Shipping and handling charges.

Total of Goods	
Shipping Charges	
Rush Charges	
Kettlebell Shipping Charges	
OH residents add 6.5% sales tax	
MN residents add 6.5% sales tax	
TOTAL ENCLOSED	

METHOD OF PAYMENT ❏ CHECK ❏ M.O. ❏ MASTERCARD ❏ VISA ❏ DISCOVER ❏ AMEX

Account No. *(Please indicate all the numbers on your credit card)*   EXPIRATION DATE

☐☐☐☐ ☐☐☐☐ ☐☐☐☐ ☐☐☐☐   ☐☐/☐☐

Day Phone: (___)_____

Signature:_____ Date:_____

NOTE: *We ship best method available for your delivery address. Foreign orders are sent by air. Credit card or International M.O. only. For* **RUSH** *processing of your order, add an additional $10.00 per address. Available on money order & charge card orders only.*

Errors and omissions excepted. Prices subject to change without notice.

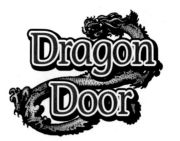

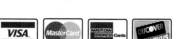

1·800·899·5111
24 HOURS A DAY • FAX YOUR ORDER (866) 280-7619
ORDERING INFORMATION

Telephone Orders For faster service you may place your orders by calling Toll Free 24 hours a day, 7 days a week, 365 days per year. When you call, please have your credit card ready.

Customer Service Questions? Please call us between 9:00am– 11:00pm EST

Monday to Friday at 1-800-899-5111. Local and foreign customers call 513-346-4160 for orders and customer service

100% One-Year Risk-Free Guarantee. If you are not completely satisfied with any product—we'll be happy to give you a prompt exchange, credit, or refund, as

you wish. Simply return your purchase to us, and please let us know why you were dissatisfied—it will help us to provide better products and services in the future. *Shipping and handling fees are non-refundable.*

Complete and mail with full payment to: Dragon Door Publications, 5 County Road B East, Suite 3, Little Canada, MN 55117

Please print clearly
Sold To: A
Name_____
Street_____
City_____
State _____ Zip _____
Day phone*_____
* Important for clarifying questions on orders

Please print clearly
SHIP TO: *(Street address for delivery)*   B
Name_____
Street_____
City_____
State _____ Zip _____
Email_____

Warning to foreign customers:
The Customs in your country may or may not tax or otherwise charge you an additional fee for goods you receive. Dragon Door Publications is charging you only for U.S. handling and international shipping. Dragon Door Publications is in no way responsible for any additional fees levied by Customs, the carrier or any other entity.

ITEM #	QTY.	ITEM DESCRIPTION	ITEM PRICE	A OR B	TOTAL

HANDLING AND SHIPPING CHARGES • NO COD'S
Total Amount of Order Add (Excludes kettlebells and kettlebell kits):

$00.00 to 29.99	Add $6.00	$100.00 to 129.99	Add $14.00
$30.00 to 49.99	Add $7.00	$130.00 to 169.99	Add $16.00
$50.00 to 69.99	Add $8.00	$170.00 to 199.99	Add $18.00
$70.00 to 99.99	Add $11.00	$200.00 to 299.99	Add $20.00
		$300.00 and up	Add $24.00

Canada and Mexico add $6.00 to US charges. All other countries, flat rate, double US Charges. See Kettlebell section for Kettlebell Shipping and handling charges.

Total of Goods	
Shipping Charges	
Rush Charges	
Kettlebell Shipping Charges	
OH residents add 6.5% sales tax	
MN residents add 6.5% sales tax	
TOTAL ENCLOSED	

METHOD OF PAYMENT ❏ CHECK ❏ M.O. ❏ MASTERCARD ❏ VISA ❏ DISCOVER ❏ AMEX
Account No. *(Please indicate all the numbers on your credit card)*   EXPIRATION DATE

▢▢▢▢ ▢▢▢▢ ▢▢▢▢ ▢▢▢▢   ▢▢/▢▢

Day Phone: (___)_____
Signature: _____ **Date:** _____

NOTE: *We ship best method available for your delivery address. Foreign orders are sent by air. Credit card or International M.O. only. For* **RUSH** *processing of your order, add an additional $10.00 per address. Available on money order & charge card orders only.*

Errors and omissions excepted. Prices subject to change without notice.

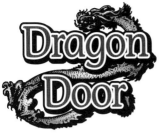

1·800·899·5111

24 HOURS A DAY • FAX YOUR ORDER (866) 280-7619

O R D E R I N G   I N F O R M A T I O N

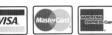 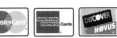

Telephone Orders For faster service you may place your orders by calling Toll Free 24 hours a day, 7 days a week, 365 days per year. When you call, please have your credit card ready.

Customer Service Questions? Please call us between 9:00am– 11:00pm EST

Monday to Friday at 1-800-899-5111. Local and foreign customers call 513-346-4160 for orders and customer service

100% One-Year Risk-Free Guarantee. If you are not completely satisfied with any product—we'll be happy to give you a prompt exchange, credit, or refund, as

you wish. Simply return your purchase to us, and please let us know why you were dissatisfied—it will help us to provide better products and services in the future. *Shipping and handling fees are non-refundable.*

Complete and mail with full payment to: Dragon Door Publications, 5 County Road B East, Suite 3, Little Canada, MN 55117

Please print clearly

Sold To: **A**

Name_____

Street _____

City _____

State _____ Zip _____

Day phone*_____
*Important for clarifying questions on orders

Please print clearly

SHIP TO: *(Street address for delivery)*   **B**

Name_____

Street _____

City _____

State _____ Zip _____

Email _____

Warning to foreign customers:
The Customs in your country may or may not tax or otherwise charge you an additional fee for goods you receive. Dragon Door Publications is charging you only for U.S. handling and international shipping. Dragon Door Publications is in no way responsible for any additional fees levied by Customs, the carrier or any other entity.

ITEM #	QTY.	ITEM DESCRIPTION	ITEM PRICE	A OR B	TOTAL

HANDLING AND SHIPPING CHARGES • NO COD'S
Total Amount of Order Add (Excludes kettlebells and kettlebell kits):

$00.00 to 29.99	Add $6.00	$100.00 to 129.99	Add $14.00
$30.00 to 49.99	Add $7.00	$130.00 to 169.99	Add $16.00
$50.00 to 69.99	Add $8.00	$170.00 to 199.99	Add $18.00
$70.00 to 99.99	Add $11.00	$200.00 to 299.99	Add $20.00
		$300.00 and up	Add $24.00

Canada and Mexico add $6.00 to US charges. All other countries, flat rate, double US Charges. See Kettlebell section for Kettlebell Shipping and handling charges.

Total of Goods	
Shipping Charges	
Rush Charges	
Kettlebell Shipping Charges	
OH residents add 6.5% sales tax	
MN residents add 6.5% sales tax	
TOTAL ENCLOSED	

METHOD OF PAYMENT ❑ CHECK ❑ M.O. ❑ MASTERCARD ❑ VISA ❑ DISCOVER ❑ AMEX

Account No. *(Please indicate all the numbers on your credit card)*   EXPIRATION DATE

☐☐☐☐ ☐☐☐☐ ☐☐☐☐ ☐☐☐☐   ☐☐/☐☐

Day Phone: (____)_____

Signature: _____   Date: _____

---

*NOTE: We ship best method available for your delivery address. Foreign orders are sent by air. Credit card or International M.O. only. For **RUSH** processing of your order, add an additional $10.00 per address. Available on money order & charge card orders only.*

Errors and omissions excepted. Prices subject to change without notice.